# Wisdom by Nature

## The New Approach to Healing Gastroparesis and Digestive Challenges

---

Chalyce Macoskey, MA, CHHC, CAC
and Stephanie Torres, CHC

Healing GP Naturally
Nokomis, Florida

This book is dedicated to those living with
gastroparesis and the people who care for them.
Never give up; there's always hope.

# Contents

CHAPTER 9

## Recipes for Healing Gastroparesis Naturally

Liquids to Assist in Digestive Support
    Himalayan Salt Sole
    Kristine's Dairy Kefir Milk
    Kristine's Water Kefir
    Miso Soup
    Golden Milk
    Nourishing Bone Broth
Easy-to-Digest Soups and Porridge
    Kitchari
    Congee
    Bieler Broth
    Journey with Gastroparesis Create-A-Soup
    Sweet Potato Cream of Rice
    Buckwheat Pumpkin Porridge
Veggie Sides
    Moroccan Spiced Sweet Potatoes
    Zucchini Ribbons and Summer Sauce
Pancakes Two Ways
    Sprouted Pancakes for Everyone
    Pumpkin Pancakes
Shared Experiences: Stephanie's Journey with Gastroparesis

The Chemistry of Essential Oils
All About Coconut Oil
Suggested Products
Online Resources
References
Acknowledgments

# Foreword

Dear Readers,

When I was first contacted by Chalyce Macoskey, owner of Essential7, I was skeptical about essential oils. Being trained and working as a medical doctor, what I had heard about essential oils was that they smell either good or bad; you can rub some on various parts of your body; and while they won't hurt or make things worse, who knows if they are really helpful.

However, considering myself an open-minded person and being offered a free sample of eight various essential oils, I decided to give them a shot.

Suffering from insomnia, I started with the Kathy's Sleep blend. To my surprise, I didn't have insomnia that first night. I used it again and again, getting the same result—a good night's sleep and no more insomnia. However, being the inquisitive skeptic, I decided to not use it for a few nights and see what would happen as maybe it was just the placebo effect. Well, big mistake, as my insomnia came right back. After a few bad nights of insomnia, I was back to applying Kathy's Sleep essential oil, sleeping very peacefully and waking well-rested each morning.

I next decided to try the Focus and Clarify blend, and again noticed that these essential oils not only worked but serve a purpose. I started using one essential oil after another from the sample of eight, testing them the same way I did Kathy's Sleep (i.e. on and off until I realized that without them my symptoms reappeared but with them I felt better.)

Immediately I requested some more samples from Chalyce to help friends who had expressed challenges ranging from excessive soreness, stomach and digestive problems, stress, anxiety and depression. The feedback I received was always the same: The oils were working and they wanted to know where they could order more.

I did some medical research and discovered other doctors throughout the world were using oils on patients with various ailments and attaining positive results. I also found published articles on the medical benefits of essential oils. So, while I started out as a skeptic, I am now proudly a spokesperson for Essential7, quite frankly because the oils work. You don't have to take just my word for it, you can also take the medical profession's word for it, as the results have been proven and published.

Dr. Joseph Krachenfels
Osteopathic and Family Medicine Physician
San Francisco, California

# About the Authors

**Chalyce Macoskey** is an IV-certified medical assistant with certifications in both aromatherapy and holistic health coaching. She is the founder and chief executive officer of Wisdom by Nature, a company that provides education for optimal wellness, and the owner of Essential7, a company that wholesales ethically produced, premium-quality essential oils to other manufacturers. Currently, she serves as the vice president of aromatherapy for the Natural Therapies Certification Board.

Chalyce is a pioneer in the use of essential oils and nutrition to assist in the overall well-being and improved quality of life for individuals of all ages. From a young age, Chalyce lived with stomach challenges and as a teenager, she was given a diagnosis that was termed "cheerleader syndrome." Nearly 30 years ago, not much was known about gastroparesis and her doctor believed her challenges stemmed from the pressure of being an active student. She later experienced IBS, fibromyalgia, uncontrolled gestational diabetes, hypoglycemia, Epstein Barr virus and autoimmune challenges. Chalyce took a variety of medications over the course of her life until, in her early 20s, a "country" doctor taught her how to start helping herself through diet, supplements and whole-food nutrition. This is where her journey to help others began.

Since starting her research in Golden, Colorado, Chalyce has extensively researched the role of natural therapies and whole-food nutrition, and now coaches clients throughout the world who face complex medical challenges. Chalyce specializes in the formulation of essential oil blends that address the issues of each individual client. Her unique approach to wellness has changed lives. She has assisted clients with conditions ranging from MRSA, antibiotic-resistant infections, as well as Stevens–Johnson Syndrome. She also specializes in coaching others in healthy ways to overcome women's health and digestive challenges.

Chalyce has an unwavering commitment to finding the right blend of essential oils and organic whole-food nutrition to bring drastic improvements in clients' conditions and quality of life. Today, Chalyce is an advocate for healing the body, mind and spirit with whole-food nutrition as well as with essential oils.

In her lectures and consulting practice, Chalyce shares that no matter their age, people can improve their quality of life by addressing root causes and healing at the cellular level. She is especially concerned with children and senior citizens, who often are faced with specific challenges not seen in the general population. She travels all over the country giving lectures and educating individuals and organizations on how to shop in a more holistic manner on a budget.

In 2013, Chalyce began to take part in the Healing Gastroparesis Naturally Facebook page, created by her friend Kathleen Atkins, to facilitate coaching of individuals dealing with GP. To date, more than 1,500 individuals have found improved quality of life via her coaching. In 2016, she completed a grant-funded study on how essential oils improve quality of life for those challenged with gastroparesis. The results are to be published in 2017 in the journal *Holistic Nursing Practice, The Science of Health and Healing.*

Chalyce believes that we can make a difference in the body's ability to overcome challenges: The key is in learning the essential principles in wellness.

**Stephanie Torres** was officially diagnosed with gastroparesis in 2008 at the age of 28, following years of digestive problems. Luckily, in her early 20s, she had found a passion for nutrition, yoga and meditation. Despite the many challenges she has faced over the years, Stephanie has continued to use these methods to help manage her illness.

Certified as a health coach in 2012 through the Institute for Integrative Nutrition, Stephanie currently works as a consumer advocate with ThriveRx, providing one-on-one support and education for those on home enteral and parenteral nutrition. Through her blog, Journey with Gastroparesis, she has shared experiences, insight and tips for living with GP. She attends conferences and support groups across the country and has helped to raise awareness and funds for research through the annual Awareness Walk for Gastroparesis & Digestive Health.

After noticing the difference essential oils made in her own life, she began working with Chalyce Macoskey and the non-profit Wisdom by Nature to help spread awareness about the use of essential oils and natural remedies for GP.

Stephanie lives with her husband and two fur babies in Washington state where she enjoys cuddling up with a good book, writing, cooking, traveling, "Netflixing" and spending time with friends and family.

# –1–
## Laying the Foundation

*"It is better to believe than to disbelieve; in so doing
you bring everything to the realm of possibility."*
-Albert Einstein

Years ago, as I was working as an IV-certified medical assistant, I had no idea how much one summer would change my life, and ultimately the lives of many others. On July 17, 2000, as I drove down a winding, Colorado mountain road, my car was struck by another vehicle.

As a result of the accident, I suffered from severe brain trauma; losing my short-term memory and cognitive thinking abilities. Reading and writing became a struggle, simply speaking was a challenge, and grocery shopping completely impossible. I was prescribed a variety of medications to help me focus, to sleep and to prevent anxiety attacks. I worked with multiple therapists to cope during my recovery. The brain injury resulted in me no longer feeling hunger; my weight dropped to an all-time low of 85 pounds. Challenged with digestive issues my whole life, this new problem was much more severe than anything I had experienced before.

During a visit to my chiropractor, I ran into an old friend. Sev-

*eral years before, the friend had introduced me to essential oils for my son's strep throat, which, to my surprise, worked wonders. My friend noticed how ill I looked and offered to help through the use of essential oils, diet modifications and homeopathy. Over the next several months, I regained my health and decided to dedicate my life to helping others do the same.*

*In 2010, I became certified as an aromatherapy coach as well as a holistic health coach. Because I combined my medical background with what I learned about nutrition from my own recovery, people began to seek help from me and my New Approach when all other medical systems were failing them.*

## What Does Healing Truly Mean?

Chalyce's experiences before this accident and following it all led to her desire to help people heal. The word "healing" can be confusing and misunderstood. When we talk about "healing" gastroparesis naturally, it may be misinterpreted as offering a cure, or can perhaps put off people who spend too much time and energy looking for answers, yet continue to suffer. Healing can come in many forms, but we take it to mean "making whole." In other words, finding balance and an improvement in quality of life when it comes to all aspects—physical, mental and spiritual.

According to Wikipedia, "In psychiatry and psychology, healing is the process by which neuroses and psychoses are resolved *to the degree that the client is able to lead a normal or fulfilling existence without being overwhelmed* by psychopathological phenomena. This process may involve psychotherapy, pharmaceutical treatment or alternative approaches such as traditional spiritual approaches." This definition offers another example of what we mean by balance and improved quality of life. To have the ability to lead a fulfilling existence could mean having enough energy to attend your child's soccer game, work at a job you feel passionate about, make nourishing meals, take a vacation, attend school and so on.

You have the ability to heal yourself to whatever degree is needed for your quality of life.

Gastroenterologist Dr. Gerard Mullin (a doctor Stephanie had the pleasure to visit at Johns Hopkins in 2012) couldn't have said it better in his book, *The Inside Tract*. "We all have the healing force within us that holds the key to our recovery," Mullin writes. "Understand that this isn't a mystical or metaphysical statement. It's not something we simply believe—it is biological reality. Your body was built to be healthy and to heal itself when illness occurs. But to take advantage of your body's inherent healing energies, you need to find balance again. In seeing countless patients over the years, we have seen the best results when the anatomy of illness is seen not only as physical ailment, but also as a matrix of imbalances in the mind, body and spirit. Recognizing this, realigning your lifestyle, and rebalancing your whole self will give you the best chance at healing."

## What Is Gastroparesis?

Gastro-what? What do you mean my stomach doesn't work? Can it be cured? Will medications help? Will I always struggle every day?

For many people with gastroparesis, these questions sound all too familiar.

Gastroparesis (GP) literally means "stomach paralysis" and is also referred to as delayed gastric emptying. When someone is healthy and the stomach functions at a normal rate, contractions of the stomach help to break up food and then move it further down the gastrointestinal tract, where continued digestion and absorption of nutrients occurs. With gastroparesis, food moves slowly or may stop moving completely from the stomach down its path to the small intestine.

This condition can result in early satiety, or feeling full with just a few bites, nausea, vomiting, abdominal pain, bloating, reflux and lack of appetite. Over time a person can become malnourished, dizzy, fatigued, and can experience unintentional weight loss or gain, body aches, erratic blood sugar levels and more. Getting out of bed in the morning can feel daunting, not to mention facing daily tasks such as going to work or school, caring for a family, driving, preparing meals and the simple things many people often take for granted.

If you are reading this book, you most likely have been diagnosed with gastroparesis (GP) or someone you love is struggling with it. Days and nights can be plagued with nausea, bloating, abdominal pain, irregular bowel movements, reflux and/or vomiting. Other challenges you may experience include fatigue, dizziness, headaches, body pain, chronic infections, anemia, malnutrition and so on. You will come to see how connected these challenges are as you continue to navigate through the following chapters. Let's begin by looking at common causes, complications and testing for gastroparesis.

## What Causes Gastroparesis?

Nobody really knows what causes GP for many of those diagnosed. One possibility is damage to the vagus nerve, an important nerve that helps control the stomach muscles and movement of food through the digestive tract. The vagus nerve can be damaged during surgery or by diseases such as diabetes. We will talk more about the wonders of this "wandering nerve" in chapter 4.

Other factors that might slow the spontaneous movement of

the stomach muscles and make it difficult to empty the stomach include: infection, such as one caused by a virus; medications that slow the rate of motility, including narcotic pain medications; certain cancer treatments like radiation therapy; scleroderma or Ehlers-Danlos syndrome (connective tissue disorders); nervous system diseases, such as Parkinson's or multiple sclerosis; and hypothyroidisms (low thyroid).

According to the National Organization for Rare Disorders, young and middle-aged women are most likely to be affected by idiopathic gastroparesis, meaning GP that has no known cause.

## Complications

Many complications can arise from chronic gastroparesis:

- **Malnutrition**: Because GP causes patients to not feel hungry, it can be a struggle to take in enough nutrients and calories or to properly absorb nutrients from food consumed. Eating may result in vomiting, or the food may not move quickly enough through the digestive system for absorption.

- **Dehydration**: May be caused by vomiting or not drinking enough water during the day due to satiety (feeling full) or other symptoms.

- **Bezoars**: Hardened masses of undigested food are sometimes found in the stomach. These masses may cause nausea and vomiting and can be life-threatening as they prevent food from passing into the small intestine.

- **Decreased quality of life**: Flare-ups can make it difficult to work and to fully participate in and enjoy life.

# Diagnosing Gastroparesis

Your doctor may order these tests:

- **Upper GI endoscopy**: The upper gastrointestinal (GI) tract is observed during this procedure, which can reveal problems that do not appear on an x-ray. The upper GI tract includes the esophagus, stomach and the first part of the small intestine called the duodenum. A tiny camera on the end of a long, flexible tube called an endoscope is inserted into the mouth and gently moved down the throat to the upper GI tract. Since the entire upper GI tract can be seen during this test, it can also be called an EGD or esophagogastroduodenoscopy. During an EGD, the doctor can check for ulcers, inflammation, tumors, infection or bleeding, and take tissue samples called a biopsy, if needed.

- **Computerized tomography (CT), enterography and magnetic resonance (MR) enterography**: A particular type of non-invasive CT imaging done with IV contrast material after ingestion of a liquid that helps produce high-resolution images of the small intestine and other structures in the pelvis and abdomen. A CT or CAT scan is a medical diagnostic test that produces multiple images of the inside of the body, like an x-ray, only more detailed.

- **Gastric emptying study (GES)**: During this test, a light meal that contains a small amount of radioactive material is consumed. A scanner is placed over the abdomen to detect the movement of the radioactive material to measure the rate food leaves the stomach over a period of two to four hours, with four hours being the most reliable. This test is the gold standard for diagnosing gastroparesis.

- **Upper GI series**: A series of x-rays is taken following the intake of barium contrast, a white, chalky liquid that can coat the digestive tract to help identify any abnormalities.

- **Gastric emptying breath test (GEBT):** Approved by the FDA in 2015, this test is conducted over a four-hour period following an overnight fast. It is designed to show how quickly the stomach empties solids by measuring carbon dioxide in a patient's breath. Patients have baseline breath tests done at the beginning of the procedure. These are followed with a special test meal that includes a scrambled egg mix with Spirulina platensis, a type of protein that has been enriched with carbon-13, which can be measured in breath samples.

Once someone is diagnosed with gastroparesis, common treatment options include dietary modifications (i.e. low-fat or low-fiber foods; smaller, more frequent meals; avoiding of raw fruits and vegetables); medications used for motility and to treat symptoms that occur such as pain, nausea and vomiting; a surgically placed gastric pacemaker; injections of botox to the stomach; feeding tubes; and IV nutrition. Some practitioners are now also recommending complementary and alternative therapies like acupuncture, cognitive behavioral therapy and lifestyle modifications.

## The New Approach

Based on her own experience with digestion challenges and in working with clients over the years, Chalyce developed what we call the New Approach, which encompasses healthy, natural alternatives. This protocol is designed to minimize your challenges and perhaps provide a new level of health in mind, body and spirit that you may have never experienced before. The New Approach is based on:

- **Changes to the diet.** When you are living with a challenging digestive disorder like GP, it is of vital importance to eat nutrient-dense food and foods that are chemical-free. Eating as "clean" as possible is equally important because added chemicals in foods may create more stress on the body. Clean eating does not mean you have to go completely organic. It is about learning how to read labels, discovering that less is more, and understanding that foods free of added hormones, steroids and antibiotics are a must when giving the body a chance to heal. You will read more about clean eating later in this book.

- **Essential oils.** Essential oils are a critical part of this regimen and will be discussed in detail throughout the book.

- **Forms of alternative therapies.** Acupuncture, Reiki, hypnosis, chanting, reflexology, meditation and yoga, journaling and energy work can all be of great benefit in supporting your mind, body and spirit.

This book includes many voices: You will hear from the authors, healthcare practitioners and fellow GP'ers of all ages. You will hear from mothers desperate to stop their children's suffering; husbands and wives who want their lives and families back; as well as many others who trust in our New Approach. Through the Shared Experiences in this book you'll hear from others who describe their digestive challenges in their own words. To read the full accounts of these contributors, please visit www.healinggpnaturally.info/healinggpbook.

You will also find journal exercises designed to help you capture your feelings, note the healing actions you take and record their outcomes. You can write your responses directly in this book, or go to www.healinggpnaturally.info/healinggpbook to download printable versions of the exercises to keep in a separate journal or notebook.

Reading this book may make you cry—with joy, with understanding, with the realization that "Yes, yes, that is me! Someone finally gets what I am saying!"

## SHARED EXPERIENCES

### Kathleen's Story: No One Gets to Take Our Hope Away

*The digestive problems began when Kathleen was in her 20s. They were a bit vague and included nausea and sometimes vomiting. During her first pregnancy, she was frequently hospitalized for dehydration and vomited constantly, even in the delivery room the day her child was born. But at the time nobody gave it much thought.*

*After her daughter was born, Kathleen learned to live with nausea. She didn't eat much and visited numerous GI specialists who all came up with the same diagnoses: irritable bowel syndrome (IBS), reflux, gastritis and esophagitis. Eventually, she stopped going to doctors. She had become tired of hearing how the only treatments were proton pump inhibitors (PPIs, or medications that reduce gastric acid production). Kathleen spent almost 30 years on PPIs, all while enduring considerable pain, nausea and vomiting.*

*At one point, Kathleen spent two years pestering GI specialists to do a gallbladder function study. The results showed that her gallbladder was functioning at just 4 percent. Six weeks later, it was removed, but the problems continued. At this point, her exasperated GI specialist informed her that "women were not equipped to be a wife, mother and a successful businesswoman," and that it "must be in her head." So, off to the shrink she went. He listened intently to all she had to say, and declared her sound of mind but certainly not of body. He did, however, recommend that she find a new GI specialist.*

*Kathleen found a female GI, hoping for some empathy, with no such luck. The first test performed was a gastric emptying study. One week later, the diagnosis of gastroparesis was introduced.*

*"How do I make it go away?" Kathleen asked. "Is it terminal?"
The doctor said matter-of-factly, "It's a chronic condition. It may
not kill you, but by the time it's done with you, you'll wish it had."*

*Kathleen asked for a specialist and was referred to allegedly the
best motility doctor in her area. Under that physician's care, she
spent the next eight years enduring a variety of tests and therapies
in an attempt to alleviate her symptoms. By the third visit, she
was told to consider the gastric stimulator, a device implanted in
the wall of the stomach to help contract the stomach muscles. Desperate, she agreed, but spent the next year suffering with electric
shocks, pain and loss of bowel control from the stimulator. None of
this balanced out the very slight improvement of her nausea and
vomiting. Exasperated, Kathleen asked to have it removed—only
then was she advised that the stimulator may only work on idiopathic GP about 10 percent of the time. A far cry from the 75
percent success rate she had been told.*

*Over the next eight years, for every symptom Kathleen experi-
enced, her doctor would throw a prescription at it. She dropped more
than 30 pounds, had insomnia and lived in a state of fear. She looked
pale and drawn. The pain was horrible. She would go to the ER only
to be told it was no place for chronic disease. At no point was nutrition mentioned. Her specialist asked her which was worse: the pain
or the inability to eat? "Why do I have to choose?" she asked.*

*Kathleen began to decline rapidly. Fortunately, a friend who
had been a respiratory therapist called her one day. Hearing her
inability to breathe, he sent an ambulance to her home. Her pulse
was faint and weak, and her blood pressure was dangerously low.
The EMT started an IV right there in her living room.*

*The ER resident didn't believe she had gone six weeks with-
out eating, even though Kathleen's husband corroborated the story.
When the labs came back, all hell broke loose. Magnesium, potassi-*

um and calcium IVs came in from every direction. The staff actually believed she was in pain and occasionally remembered to give her a pain pill without her asking. In the hospital, she lost five more pounds, but passed two psychiatric evaluations, was prescribed a narcotic pain reliever, and given a "quality of life over quantity of life" speech. She chose not to fill the prescription. Frightened but determined, she went home.

Kathleen called Lynette, a close friend who knew Chalyce Macoskey, a holistic health and aromatherapy coach. Soon Chalyce flew to Kathleen's home and immediately began coaching Kathleen on how to apply a combination of essential oils every hour she could stay awake. Kathleen learned to support her stomach with Latta Kefir and began eating nutrient-dense food within 12 hours of Chalyce's arrival. That was in October 2013.

Today, Kathleen follows the New Approach as much as possible. There are days when she isn't perfect, eating foods outside of what works best for her body. However, she now experiences better days and controls her challenges using natural resources. No more lists of medications, no more trips to the ER and no more doctors accusing her of being a drug seeker. Her improving health is a testament to the theories Chalyce shares about healing GP naturally. Kathleen describes her results this way:

"I am nearly done with pharmaceuticals as I continue to wean off one last medication. I use planking exercises to strengthen my core muscles, chanting to ask for healing, my wonderful essential oils, clean eating and a healthy mindset of hope to keep me focused on my goals to beat gastroparesis and the other digestive tract disorders I have lived with. No one gets to take our hope away. This is my story and I write a new page every day. Thank goodness for that; 20 years is a long time and this has been one hell of a roller coaster ride."

You may read stories such as this one and think that could never be you or can't possibly be true. Some of you are very, very sick. In fact, Stephanie is living with the help of TPN (IV nutrition through a port in her chest) while she focuses on the New Approach to help manage discomfort and increase her food intake. But, for the first time in years, she has been able to eat more without immediate pain and have a quality of life she didn't think was possible. Wherever you are, we want to help you improve your life.

Unlike traditional medicine that focuses on symptoms, with the New Approach we explore the reason the symptoms have come to be. We believe when you support the body, it has *the best* ability to heal itself. Traditional medicine has its place in many situations, from acute care to life-saving events. Advances in medical technology are incredible and continue to save lives every day. But for challenges such as GP and digestive distress, a different approach should be explored as well, because there are not always enough answers for chronic challenges in traditional medicine.

When you have GP, your body is in a state of dis-ease, something is off balance and homeostasis no longer exists. In Chalyce's experience and research, she has found that an unbalanced body becomes acidic, which can then create an environment that allows GP and other conditions such as heart disease, high blood pressure, diabetes and cancer to grow. Through education, you can begin to take steps to improve your quality of life. Educate yourself on the things that support the body and prevent more dis-ease. You are doing that right here, right now. No matter the health challenge, the steps are the same: Support the body through the right nutrition, the right therapies (essential oils, meditation, yoga, etc.), and the right supplements.

Let's begin to improve your quality of life!

## Journal Exercise: Script to Self

Begin a journal of your journey to health. This journal can take any form you choose. Write in a spiral-bound notebook or go to the store and spend a little bit of time finding a journal with a cover that more personally represents your journey, that brings you joy and inspiration.

On the inside, starting with page one, please write:

I, _____ (your name) agree on this _____ day of 20___ to rewrite my life script around gastroparesis and to arrive at a healthy, happy, improved level of health and nutrition. I realize that I will need to be honest with myself about many areas of my life. I embrace this new path of life with open arms for I have nothing to lose and everything to gain. I know that I am not alone on this journey, and I will remember to ask for help when I need it and to reach out to those who support me whenever I need to be reminded of this. I am excited to step onto this new path filled with hope.

Signed: _____

Date:_____

## AFFIRMATION

*I am healthy in mind, body and spirit and I can accomplish anything I put my mind to.*

# −2−
## Healing and Essential Oils:
## A Different Way of Thinking

*"The eye sees only what the mind is prepared to comprehend."*
-Henri Bergson

It takes patience and practice to have on open mind. It means embracing new ideas, possibilities and suggestions. If you have dealt with illness for a long time, your patience has most likely been tested in every way possible by doctors, exams, treatments and even family and friends. Our goal is not to make you more fearful, but to provide an approach that will give you hope and, like so many others we have worked with, a much improved quality of life!

Health information is everywhere: on the news, in commercials, magazines and on the internet. It sometimes comes from well-meaning family and friends who share what they think is in your best interest. Many who suffer with chronic illness also look for the answers themselves, a search that can be frustrating. Numerous Western medications will treat the challenges of GP but may not remedy the illness itself. While medications have their place, the research done for this book and our experience shows there are many alternative aids for those living with a chronic condition such as GP.

Many of you are discouraged by some of your doctors and their responses to your questions. They may not have answers or the key to the mysteries that lie beneath this incurable disorder. Unfortunately, doctors do not always have the education they should on nutrition. In the Medscape article, "Doctors Need to Learn More About Nutrition," Dr. Stephen R. Devries shares, "I know from my own training 25 years ago, I received essentially no education in nutrition in three years of an internal medicine residency and four years of cardiovascular fellowship training." Despite the knowledge gained in the interim about the link between nutrition and health, very little has changed regarding nutrition education in the past 25 years. We should not fault the medical profession for that, but instead, we should help educate and inspire practitioners to want to know more about supporting the body as a whole, which at times can lead to healing. This knowledge of nutrition is the key to improving quality of life for people with chronic illness.

There was a time when "country" doctors were the ones that offered natural, homeopathic remedies first, often using Western medication as a last resort. They advised their patients that medication was not always a cure, and might have suggested that their patients stop smoking so much or cut back on sweets, or exercise and get plenty of rest.

In today's fast-paced society we have come to expect a quick fix. We now have the pharmaceutical companies supplying our demand. We have forgotten that an apple a day keeps the doctor away, so to speak. We go to our medicine cabinet and grab the quickest fix for heartburn, acid reflux, headaches, colds and the flu. You name it, for many acute health problems, there is a medication to treat it quickly. But when it comes to chronic illness, while there may be medications, procedures and therapies to help, where do we go from there? What has happened to us? We are the sickest we have ever been. Why? Because most medicine often chooses to take the easy way out, to help us temporarily feel better, or to just simply survive. But do we feel better in the long-term? No, because we have abused medications for their easy fix. And when a person with GP experiences so much pain and suffering, it is understandable to want an answer and to want it fast. "I can't and will not wait; I have a life!" But by thinking this short-term way we have lost our quality of life.

What we share here are ideas for improving quality of life by giving the body what it needs to heal itself, not focusing simply on treating the symptoms.

Remember healing literally means to make whole; to find balance and an improvement in quality of life—a process that takes time.

## SHARED EXPERIENCES

### Kate's Story: Hope and Inspiration

*Meet Kate, born in 1996, who at the age of 3 developed cyclic vomiting syndrome (CVS). Going to the emergency room became normal for Kate and between the ages of 6 and 8, she became slower to bounce back from episodes. A gastroenterologist informed the family that Kate would not outgrow CVS and suggested that stress could be contributing.*

*Between the ages of 10 and 13, Kate's episodes increased, followed by the need for lengthy infusions of IV fluids. She now suffered from headaches, nausea and abdominal pain. In addition, she went through toxic shock syndrome that landed her in the hospital with sepsis. Numerous tests were done, with results that continued to come back as normal, negative or non-conclusive. Kate's* weight dropped to 81 pounds and she missed 45 days of her 8th grade school year.

Kate's medication list was long: a proton pump inhibitor, an anti-nauseant, an opioid painkiller and more. She was referred to an eating disorder specialist, who did not believe Kate suffered from an eating disorder, but rather from "disordered eating due to never being able to digest food!"

In November 2011, Kate's mother contacted Chalyce Macoskey through a mutual friend. Following a Skype session, Chalyce made immediate travel plans and carefully handcrafted a unique personal regimen of care to slowly rebuild Kate's delicate body and spirit. The regimen included selected essential oils applied to the soles of Kate's feet throughout the day, a nutrient-rich diet of small meals every two hours, magnesium and other remedies that would soon bring her health back. Chalyce even created a special oil blend for her use called Kate's Happy Tummy.

Kate's mom sums it all up: "Today Kate maintains a healthy weight, restored muscle tone and strength, exceeds in AP level classes, resumed an active lifestyle and has traveled and been able to restore valuable friendships." Her goal is to attend university in the fall and pursue a career in the medical field aimed at helping children.

## Getting Started: The Basics

Please keep in mind the information and ideas being shared here are only suggestions. Everyone is different, and some suggestions may not work for you. You know your body best and will learn to make adjustments that are optimal for your needs. Remember, this is a process: Rushing it will only discourage you. Positive affirmations, chanting and short meditations are very powerful tools that are part of our New Approach.

The next few chapters of this book explain all the elements

of the New Approach and the rationale and research behind them. If you'd like to start the protocol right away, you can skip ahead to chapter 5, Putting It All Together, then return to read this background material later.

Let's start here with the wonderful world of essential oils, and those specifically created for GP.

## Using Essential Oils

Essential oils are primarily the life essence of a plant. The fragrant, highly concentrated liquid is commonly created through steam distilling the petals, stems, leaves, barks, roots or other elements of the plant.

Essential oils can be inhaled, or absorbed by rubbing on the skin, allowing the chemical compounds that make up the composition to cross into the bloodstream. In doing so, they can improve the quality of life by creating a hostile environment for bacteria and viruses, offering pain management, optimizing performance, helping to reduce stress and even offering personal first aid.

In this book, we refer to the oils created by Essential7, a company that focuses on oils that specifically benefit digestive challenges such as gastroparesis, and whose mission is to supply the finest, purest, high-quality products. Beneficial essential oils or blends for digestive challenges include Essential7's GP Starter Collection, GP Female Support and the GP Travel Collection.

The following chart introduces you to oils and their safe application. You can photocopy this chart and place it in your journal for easy reference. Be sure to mix any essential oil that is neat (undiluted) with a carrier oil such as coconut, grapeseed, jojoba or olive oil. The suggested ratio is 4 to 5 drops of essential oil to 15 drops of carrier oil.

| ESSENTIAL OIL | BEST FOR | HOW AND WHEN | NOTES |
|---|---|---|---|
| **Clary Sage** | Female challenges | Mix 4-5 drops with 4-5 drops of carrier oil, apply to stomach area or apply neat to bottoms of feet, every 2 hours until challenges improve then upon waking and bedtime. | You may try using clary sage one week before your cycle. Once you feel in balance only use as needed not every day. |
| **Copaiba** | Challenges with stomach, diarrhea | Mix with 4-5 drops of carrier oil, apply to stomach area or apply neat to bottoms of feet, every 2 hours until challenges improve, then upon waking and bedtime. | |
| **Deep Comfort** | Female challenges or body discomfort | You may apply 4-5 drops to stomach area or apply 4-5 drops neat to bottoms of feet, every 2 hours until challenges improve, then upon waking and bedtime. | May be used daily to improve quality of your life. Then as desired |
| **Gastro**  Blend of Red Mandarin, Juniper Berry, Patchouli, Ginger Root, Aniseed, Tarragon, Peppermint | Designed for digestion support and one you will want to use for ongoing support. | Apply 4-5 drops to bottoms of feet upon waking up, before meals, bedtime | Suggested to use every hour in the beginning to feel improvement |
| **Kate's Happy Tummy**  Blend of Peppermint, Black Pepper, Spearmint | Compliments Gastro. Supports the stomach. This is your go-to when having distress after meals | Apply 4-5 drops to bottoms of feet upon waking up, before meals, bedtime | Suggested to use every hour in the beginning to feel improvement |
| **Kathy's Sleep Easy**  Blend of Labdanum, Roman Chamomile, Valerian Root, Lavender Bulgarian, Rue | Challenges related to sleep | You may apply 4-5 drops to bottoms of feet, to shirt or to pillowcase at bedtime. | Can be applied in times of extreme stress |

| ESSENTIAL OIL | BEST FOR | HOW AND WHEN | NOTES |
|---|---|---|---|
| **Quease Go Away**<br><br>Blend of Red Mandarin, Cumin, Coriander, Patchouli | Queasiness, upset stomach | Simply inhale or apply 4-5 drops to bottoms of feet when challenges occur. Every 30 minuets to an hour when needed. | |
| **Patchouli** | May reduce gastric muscle spasms, queasiness | You may apply 4-5 drops when extremely challenged. You may also try 1 drop of turmeric to wrist, rub together. Repeat with 1 drop of patchouli. | May be combined with turmeric for additonal support in times of upset. |
| **Relax and Release**<br><br>Blend of Neroli, Ylang Ylang, Patchouli, Blue Tansy, Orange 5 Fold, Tangerine | When feeling overwhelmed | Simply inhale, apply 3-4 drops to bottoms of feet or 1-2 drops to wrists. | Suggested when feeling stress or upset. May use at bedtime. |
| **Sore No More** | Female challenges or body discomfort | You may apply 4-5 drops to stomach area or apply neat to bottoms of feet, every 2 hours until challenges improve, then upon waking and bedtime. | May be used daily to improve quality of your life. Then as desired. |
| **Turmeric** | Bloating, digestive challenges | Mix with 4-5 drops of carrier oil, apply to stomach area or apply neat to bottoms of feet, every 30 minutes until challenges improve then upon waking and bedtime. | If rash occurs on stomach only apply to bottoms of feet. |

If you are pregnant or are using oils with children under the age of 2, please check with your healthcare practitioner and a certified aromatherapy coach about safe practices.

The following are suggestions to use in the beginning of the healing process to help improve quality of life. As you use the blends, you will begin to find, in time, when and how often each of them works best for your challenges.

As you start following the New Approach, you may try massaging 4 to 5 drops of an oil into the sole of each foot every two hours until you feel you have achieved your goal with the digestive challenge. Once you begin to feel more comfortable, you may then try applying 4 or 5 drops of Kate's Happy Tummy to the bottoms of feet in the morning, at noon and in the evening, and 4 or 5 drops of Gastro blend to the same area before eating. These applications alone may improve your quality of life with digestion.

You may also try turmeric oil on the bottoms of feet in the morning and at night, or as desired, for challenges with bloating and nausea.

- **Gastro:** You may try applying 4 or 5 drops of this blend on the bottom of each foot in the morning, before each meal and at bedtime if desired.

- **Kate's Happy Tummy:** 4 or 5 drops on the bottom of each foot is suggested in the morning, before each meal and at bedtime if desired.

- **Quease Go Away:** When challenged with queasiness, you may try inhaling or applying 4 or 5 drops of this blend to the bottom of each foot until you have reached your desired effect. Some have found it beneficial to apply every 30 minutes to an hour until quality of life improves.

- **Turmeric essential oil:** Experience with past clients has shown that turmeric essential oil is helpful with many digestive disorders and more specifically with bloating. You may try applying 4 or 5 drops of this essential oil mixed with 15 drops of carrier oil onto your stomach or apply neat to the bottoms of feet as needed, as often as every 30 minutes until the challenge has improved. Turmeric essential oil has been found to be very beneficial with bloating or queasiness. If a rash occurs on the stomach area, apply to the feet only.

- **Patchouli and turmeric essential oils:** Patchouli contains constituents that support digestive challenges by reducing gastrointestinal muscle contractions. To calm an upset stomach, you may try applying a drop of turmeric oil onto your wrist, then rub the wrists together. Wait one minute and do the same with one drop of patchouli oil.

- **Relax and Release:** This wonderful blend is great when you feel challenged or overwhelmed. You may inhale from the bottle, or you may try applying 3 or 4 drops on the bottom of feet or 1 or 2 drops on the wrist if desired. As time goes on you will find that your desire for the blend may become less and less as your emotions come into balance.

- **Kathy's Sleep Easy:** This blend may be beneficial for challenges related to sleep. You may try applying 4 or 5 drops on each foot before bed or placing a few drops on your shirt or pillowcase. This blend was created for Kathleen when she was dealing with trouble sleeping. (See Kathleen's story on page 15.)

- **Copaiba.** Copaiba essential oil may be beneficial for challenges with diarrhea and the stomach. You may mix 4 or 5 drops with another 15 drops of a carrier oil and apply to the stomach area or apply neat (as is) to the bottoms of feet, every two hours until challenges improve, then upon waking and at bedtime.

**What to do if you put the oils on the wrong area:** When using essential oils, if you apply the wrong one or it becomes uncomfortable, do not rinse with water but instead use a carrier oil such as coconut, olive, jojoba or almond oil. **Water and oil do not mix; *always* use another oil to remove an unwanted oil.**

Some high-grade, chemical-free essential oils are warming and you may experience discomfort if the oil is accidentally applied to an open cut or scrape. Apply the carrier oil to the site to calm discomfort quickly.

**NEVER flush with water.**

## Aromatherapy for Digestion

When we talk about essential oils and digestion, it's helpful to consider why so many cultures have used spices in cooking for centuries. We tend to think of spices as a flavor component, to make food taste good. Based on years of research and a knowledge of how herbs support digestion, spices are not all about flavor: The right herbs can support digestion and improve quality of life. In the book *Healing Spices,* the author Bharat B. Aggarwal shares that "spices contain an abundance of phytonutrients, plant compounds that bestow health and promote healing in a variety of ways."

Look at cultures all over the world: Each spice that they add to their dishes serves a purpose. Aromatic usage is just as important as ingesting the herb itself. If you think about it, when something smells good, your mouth waters and the process of digestion begins. In addition, certain aromas can trigger pleasant thoughts, which help to ease tension and anxiety.

When considering the use of herbs, keep in mind that over the years, many herbs have been superheated or highly processed. They are often grown with the use of herbicides and pesticides. This can limit their ability to do their job of supporting digestion.

Choosing organic herbs is important. Though we know organic sourcing may not always be perfect, it is the best way to limit the chemicals that enter your body.

You will find some of these herbs and spices used to help support digestion in the recipes shared in chapter 9.

The essential oils derived from some of the following herbs and spices can support digestive health and are used in Essential7 GP blends, like Gastro and Kate's Happy Tummy.

- **Peppermint.** According to the University of Maryland Medical Center (UMMC), peppermint calms the muscles of the stomach and improves the flow of bile, which the body uses to digest fats. As a result, food passes through the stomach more quickly and can allow painful digestive gas to pass. If you are challenged with frequent nausea, diarrhea or menstrual cramps, migraines, or suffer from bowel problems, peppermint oil may also be beneficial.

- **Red mandarin.** According to Organicfacts.net, "Red mandarin facilitates digestion by stimulating the discharge of digestive juices and bile into the stomach." It may also help to increase the appetite and has proved beneficial with challenges involving stomach cramps, indigestion, constipation, depression, anxiety, grief and nervousness. This oil can be used to help support digestion.

- **Ginger.** Ginger has been discovered to be a facilitator of the digestive process. Elevated sugar levels after a meal may cause the stomach to reduce its natural rate of emptying its contents. Ginger may help in regulating high sugar levels that may disrupt digestion. It can also soothe the stomach, maintaining its regular rhythm and has compounds that help improve the absorption of nutrients and minerals from food. Ginger is perfect for use as an appetizer or aperitif, since it can stimulate the appetite while also preparing the digestive system for an influx of food.

- **Cumin.** Cumin oil may promote the discharge of bile and gastric juices, and stimulate the peristaltic motion of the intestines. Its aroma acts to stimulate the appetite.

- **Coriander.** Coriander oil may improve appetite and help with challenges of nausea and vomiting. It may relieve indigestion and flatulence, and its aroma may stimulate the appetite.

## SHARED EXPERIENCES

### Lorretta's Story: Relief and Renewed Energy

*For those of you who are challenged right now, I'm sharing this to give you hope in using the New Approach.*

*I joined the Healing Gastroparesis Naturally Facebook group in late 2013 when I was pregnant with my daughter. My doctors had left me with no hope, and I was desperate for a turnaround. I was losing weight and the doctors were suggesting that I deliver the baby early. That was far from an option for me as I loved my daughter already so much. She depended on me to not only nourish myself but to provide nourishment for her as well. Doctors say she would have taken what she needed from me anyway, but her robbing me of what little I did have left me with almost nothing. I was unsure what to do. When I saw how positive and helpful everyone in the Facebook group was when I joined, I felt like this was the direction God had guided me.*

*Fast forward, starting the New Approach protocol and changing what I ate little by little, I saw progress. Sure, I had rough patches where I had to start back from the beginning, but it was a learning process and something I was willing to hang on to. When*

I got knocked back, I did not dwell on it, instead just picked myself back up and kept going.

In my first year following the New Approach, I still struggled to tolerate even the cleanest foods. I was able to add things in month by month, with the exception of all meat besides chicken, even when organic. Jumping ahead to 2016, two and a half years in to following the New Approach, one night my significant other brought home a roast beef dinner from Trader Joe's. I told him I would just eat the sides since every time I tried to eat red meat, it didn't sit well.

"What's the worst that can happen?" he asked. "You have your oils and you definitely look way better than you did a year ago." My oldest son said, "Oh come on, just a bite and if it hurts, we won't ask again." I felt defeated in a way but didn't want to disappoint these two biggest cheerleaders in my life.

Eating that meat was a gamble and I thought for sure I would regret it, but my mom taught me to always try. Life comes with many challenges, but if we never go for what we want, we will always be left wondering "what if." (Please note that I'm not suggesting anyone should be pushed into trying any food—but as you follow the New Approach you begin to know your body and what it can handle over time.)

So, I sat at the dinner table that Friday night and tried some of the beef roast, potatoes and carrots, and a nice portion as well. My family watched, ready for whatever was to come. Would I be sick, would I tolerate it? And then… I felt fine, even hours later. I thought for sure Saturday morning I would wake up with miserable nausea or pain, but I didn't. Saturday night… still okay! The look on my family's faces was filled with joy. Sunday arrived. After holding my breath for what seemed like an eternity, I knew I was going to be OK. By Monday morning, I still felt great. No symptoms, no side effects… nothing but wet eyes while writing this down!

*With this protocol comes a huge change, and it is not an over-night thing. After almost three years in, my body feels a sense of relief. I don't feel as run down; I have more energy for being a mom, passing my classes and earning my associate's degree, some-thing I thought would likely never happen.*

*I even had a surprise pregnancy a year after delivering my daughter and doctors were amazed at how much of a champ I was, given the struggles I had experienced in the past. I had rough points, but hospital visits were slim to none. I was able to enjoy every moment of it. My son was far from planned, but now I would feel incomplete without him.*

*So for those of you who are starting out: Remain positive. For those who are unsure: Go for it! And to those who have hopes of getting pregnant but have been told it is too dangerous, or who are too scared: There is hope. When your body starts to heal, or gets a break from the health challenges, you will be amazed at what you can do. Recently, my insurance company sent me a letter that said, "Congratulations, you have successfully been removed from our lock-in program!" The lock-in program is for those who receive state Medicaid or have received it and used the emergency room or visits to the doctor too much. I have not been to the ER to manage GP in who knows how long, with my last hospital stay being for the deliv-ery of my son. I have not seen my primary care physician in over a year and am not currently under the care of any specialists.*

*Am I cured? No. However, GP will not defeat me, and the more it kicks, the more I fight back. You can bet that I feel like me again. I still have a road ahead and I may fall, but I won't let it get me down.*

## AFFIRMATION

*"I will remember to be kind, compassionate and love myself first."*

# –3–
## New Foods for a New You

---

*"The doctor of the future will no longer treat the
human frame with drugs, but rather will cure and
prevent disease with nutrition."*
–Thomas Edison

This chapter focuses on the New Approach's food suggestions and the research behind those suggestions. We hope to make it easier to understand how to incorporate these lifestyle changes and how they can significantly improve your quality of life.

At first, this list of foods may seem overwhelming or contrary to what you have been told. You may be nervous to try techniques that are unfamiliar. However, once you take the time to read through this chapter, you will better understand how new food choices can truly help you.

We will first discuss traditional foods that have been around for centuries and can help the digestive tract begin to thrive. Suggestions include kefir, sauerkraut juice, Himalayan salt, coconut water and a few others. These foods have helped many people struggling with GP and other digestive challenges. Read on for suggestions on how to slowly incorporate them into your own life.

## Supportive Liquids

### Kefir

Supporting your digestion is crucial to the success of our New Approach. Begin with kefir, a type of fermented milk that originated in the Caucasus Mountains of Russia and has been a staple for many centuries. Some stories say kefir was created from goat's milk by accident. Accident or not, people felt better when they drank it and when something helps, it's worth keeping around!

Look for kefir at health food and grocery stores. Kefir made from milk from grass-fed cows is ideal, but if it's not available, purchase organic if possible. Latta Kefir is one brand we suggest. Another option as a substitute for kefir is White Mountain Bulgarian Whole Milk yogurt. In a pinch, plain Stonyfield Organic Greek Whole Fat Yogurt can be beneficial for some. It includes the culture L. Bulgaricus, also found in kefir, that supports lactic acid in the intestines (more on that soon) and is high in protein.

You might be concerned about the fat content of the foods mentioned above, but avoiding fats is not recommended. Instead, focus on taking in small amounts of fat throughout the day. For example, one cup of whole milk kefir contains approximately 8 grams of fat. When you start by consuming 1 or 2 ounces at a time, you are only taking in 1 or 2 grams of fat. According to the author of the University of Virginia's Diet Intervention for Gastroparesis, "Although fat may slow stomach emptying in some patients, many can consume fat especially in the form of liquids. Although many clinicians restrict fat, my experience is that fat in the liquid form (as part of beverages such as whole milk, milkshakes, nutritional supplements, etc.) can be well-tolerated by many. To take fat out of the diet of a patient that is seriously malnourished is to remove a valuable source of calories."

As you begin the New Approach, you may try 1 to 2 ounces of kefir every two hours or a couple of tablespoons of the Bulgarian or Stonyfield yogurt every two hours. As your stomach becomes better able to tolerate more foods, you may only need to try kefir or yogurt once a day.

Remember you are in control of what is best for you.

If you are unable to digest milk products, you may try "water grains" to create your own kefir at home. You may find kefir grains at health food stores or online that include instructions on how to start a batch. Online suppliers are listed at the end of this book. Coconut milk or coconut water can also be used as a non-dairy kefir alternative.

If you are lactose intolerant, note that most kefir brands carried in stores are labeled lactose-free. These kefirs are lactose-free due to lacto-fermentation during which the lactic-acid producing bacteria begins digesting or breaking down both milk sugar (lactose) and milk protein (casein). According to the *Handbook of Fermented Functional Foods*, by Edward R. Farnworth, "Simply put, lacto-fermentation is a microbial process using beneficial bacteria including Lactobacillus and Bifidobacterium spp. and other lactic acid bacteria (LAB) (commonly known as probiotics), which thrive in an anaerobic fermenting environment. Culturing also restores many enzymes destroyed through pasteurization. These enzymes help the body absorb calcium and other minerals. Some people, however, may simply not tolerate the dairy either due to a milk protein allergy or the current condition of their digestive system.

Although kefir must be kept refrigerated, we suggest not drinking or eating items that are cold. In Chinese medicine, the theory holds that ingesting food and beverages that are cold can slow digestion and decrease the "spleen energy." In other words, cold foods and drink can make our bodies work harder to process. If you are already challenged with slow digestion, cold food and drink may be something to avoid. Allow your kefir to get to room temperature and sip slowly.

## Sauerkraut Juice

Sauerkraut has been used in Europe for centuries to treat stomach ulcers, and numerous studies have well established its effectiveness for soothing the digestive tract. Raw sauerkraut is distinctly different from store-bought, canned sauerkraut. While many food manufacturers process their kraut using heat to extend shelf life, raw sauerkraut is lacto-fermented and is alive with good bacteria and probiotics. Raw sauerkraut is fermented over days or weeks at room temperature, packaged into jars with its own brine solution, then refrigerated to preserve the vitamins, enzymes and beneficial bacteria without any heat. The lactic acid creates beneficial intestinal flora, balances stomach acid, and helps break down proteins.

Sauerkraut juice has been used for many years in supporting digestive challenges. Some people are unable to drink sauerkraut juice because of the taste factor or because they have thyroid problems. There are concerns of goitrogens found in cruciferous vegetables, which, when consumed in large amounts, can create challenges with the thyroid itself and iodine uptake with the thyroid hormone. This is the reason for suggesting it as a condiment to support the body.

On the website Nourished and Nurtured, it is shared that fermented foods are wonderful in that they provide probiotics and nutrients, but when it comes to fermented cruciferous vegetables like sauerkraut, *moderation is key*. It is best to ensure that fermented cruciferous vegetables are consumed as condiments, not as large components of the diet. Again, the idea is to support the body and not create an imbalance by eating too much of one thing, or making problem-increasing eating choices.

*Always listen to your body.*

If a food suggestion does not seem right for you, then it probably is not.

It is suggested to try 1 teaspoon of sauerkraut juice, not the kraut itself, 20 minutes before a meal once a day to start. Try this for a few days, and then you may want to try to increase to three times a day before each meal to improve quality of life. Clients have fluctuated between a teaspoon and a tablespoon in the beginning, depending on what they are comfortable with.

For maintenance, you may try a teaspoon once or twice a week depending on your level of wellness and where you wish to be. When making these small changes, it can be common for some people to experience a little discomfort at first such as bloating or gas. Don't be concerned; you will find suggestions later in the book for addressing bloating and gas.

## Raw Apple Cider Vinegar

You might also try adding ½ teaspoon of raw apple cider vinegar to about 4 ounces of water. Take sips of the mixture 20 to 30 minutes before a meal to support intestinal flora. Bragg's Raw Apple Cider Vinegar is one product we suggest.

## Bone Broth

*"Good broth will resurrect the dead."*
–South American proverb

While packaged broth might be convenient and good for flavor, it does not contribute much when it comes to whole-food nutrition. Long-simmered stocks are typically made from the bones of chicken or beef. They can be an essential part of our diet, nourishing not only to the soul, but our entire being. For centuries, cultures all over the world have used this basic remedy to help with hundreds of diseases and ailments. As they say, chicken soup is grandma's penicillin.

Among its many attributes, broth:

- Provides easy-to-consume nutrients that can help to digest and absorb calcium, magnesium, phosphorus and other trace minerals such as sodium and potassium
- Is rich in gelatin, which may help to heal and coat the GI tract, in time improving body weight and bone density
- Contains glucosamine and chondroitin, shown to assist in reducing arthritis and joint pain
- Is rich in glycine, an amino acid that enhances gastric acid secretion. In addition, glycine detoxifies the liver, is necessary for pregnancy, and aids in recovery from malnutrition
- Facilitates digestion and absorption of proteins
- Provides soft-tissue and wound healing, healthy connective tissue and immune support.

It is suggested to sip on bone broth daily when possible or use it in your cooking. Broth can add loads of flavor to dishes like soups, kitchari, congee and pureed vegetables. Many find it comforting to sip on like a warm tea, especially during cooler weather.

## The Good Acids

### Lactic Acid

If you are challenged by the fluids mentioned above, you might try Lactic Acid Yeast Wafers by Standard Process. Do not be put off by the word yeast; the wafers will not give you yeast infections or cause more yeast in your body. The yeast is created through a fermentation process and will only support you, not create more challenges.

What is lactic acid and isn't that something bad? Well, yes and no.

Yes, in that we don't want the lactic acid that creates pain in muscles. However, lactic acid in the intestines is something completely different. It is normal bacteria that is found in the GI tract, and part of its purpose is to promote immune function. Lactic acid bacteria with Lactobacillus and Bifidobacterium creates lactic acid from carbohydrates, which are broken down through fermentation. The reason we suggest kefir, sauerkraut or raw apple cider vinegar is because they have been known to lower the pH in the GI tract and that is what we want. Lower pH may help to prevent certain infections that can create havoc in the digestion and elimination process. Lactic acid also protects the integrity of the intestinal wall and by doing so, helps to maintain good intestinal bacteria and support nutrient absorption, which is critical when you have digestive challenges.

Many people with GP are not able to absorb nutrients, making it difficult to maintain their weight and sustain quality of life. In a PubMed study released in 2006, *Probiotics and Their Fermented Food Products are Beneficial for Health*, it is suggested that "lactic acid can be involved in (i) improving intestinal tract health; (ii) enhancing the immune system, synthesizing and enhancing the bioavailability of nutrients; (iii) reducing symptoms of lactose intolerance, decreasing the prevalence of allergy in susceptible individuals; and (iv) reducing risk of certain cancers." And according to *Nourishing Traditions* author Sally Fallon, lacto-fermented foods normalize the acidity of the stomach. "If stomach acidity is insufficient, it stimulates the acid-producing glands of the stomach, and in the cases where acidity is too high it has the inverse effect."

Slowly implementing these supplements into your day can improve your quality of life.

## HCL (Stomach Acid)

HCL, or stomach acid, is good for you. Yes, you read that correctly!

Contrary to what you may have been told, stomach acid is critical for proper digestion, so we want to make sure that acid is plentiful and strong. Without enough HCL (hydrochloric acid), food cannot be completely digested in the stomach, leading to an array of health complications, including GERD, heartburn and indigestion, not to mention mineral and vitamin deficiencies.

When a person begins to eat, the chewing action alone signals the stomach to begin producing HCL, activating protein-digesting enzymes necessary for the major breakdown of food. An acidic environment is necessary for the digestive process to take place and for the food to keep moving to the small intestine. There, in a less acidic environment, food is broken down further, and important vitamins and minerals like calcium, zinc, iron, folate and B12 are absorbed. When HCL isn't strong enough, or there is not enough of it available, food stays in the stomach longer than it should, creating symptoms you may be familiar with such as bloating, gas, reflux and discomfort.

Low stomach acid can be caused by:

- Aging
- Chronic illness
- Yeast overgrowth
- Adrenal fatigue
- Bacterial infection

- Poor food combinations
- Eating a nutritionally deficient diet of processed foods, refined sugar and fast foods
- Chronic stress: HCL can be inhibited by worry and long-term stress
- Use of antacids and medications that suppress HCL production
- Vitamin and mineral deficiencies, particularly zinc and thiamine

To increase HCL production simply and gently:

- Slowly introduce fermented foods such as kefir, yogurt, sauerkraut juice and miso when starting the New Approach
- Include nutrient-dense foods and Himalayan salt
- Relax at mealtimes; for example, take five deep breaths before eating and list three things you are grateful for
- Reduce stress throughout the day with deep breathing, essential oils and mantras
- Chew, chew, chew! A good starting point is to chew at least 20 times per bite
- Stop eating at bedtime, allowing time for rest and digestion. Once you are back in balance and can go longer periods of time before eating, you may reintroduce nighttime snacks, but make sure to limit heavy snacks or eating after 7 p.m.

## Himalayan Salt

Only a certain amount of food can be digested by our intestines. If we overeat or eat improper food, our body reacts with disorder or indigestion. Using the right salt can aid in digestion by stimulating the glands that produce the digestive juices responsible for a healthy digestion. Himalayan salt stimulates hydrochloric acid and an enzyme in the stomach that comes from glands in the stomach lining. Both HCL and the enzyme digest protein and break down food while stimulating the intestinal tract and liver, which aids in the digestive process.

The following information can be found, along with a significant amount of scientific research, in Dr. Joseph Mercola's article "Add Salt to Your Food Daily" on his website, Mercola.com.

When sodium is too low, it can cause a condition known as hyponatremia. "Changes in mood and appetite are among the first noticeable manifestations of sodium deficiency, yet the cause is often missed." It can also present the following:

- Nausea and vomiting
- Loss of energy
- Muscle weakness, spasms or cramps
- Headache
- Fatigue
- Confusion
- Urinary incontinence
- Nervousness, restlessness and irritability
- Seizures

One of the important factors of Himalayan salt is that it is only 85 percent sodium chloride, compared to the 98 percent in processed table salt, with the remaining 15 percent containing 84 trace minerals from our ancient seas. Natural crystal salt supports a healthy balance in the body, helping to maintain bone health and regulate blood pressure, carrying nutrients into and out of your cells, helping your brain communicate with your muscles, and increasing brain cells associated with creativity and long-term planning.

It is suggested to use Himalayan salt, as it is an indispensable and ideal food addition in everybody's diet.

## Coconut Water and Coconut Oil

The following shared experience led to a discovery of the healing potential of coconut water and coconut oil. The following story shows the healing properties of coconut oil that truly saved the life of a dear friend who had been compromised by disease and left without hope from Western medicine.

### SHARED EXPERIENCES

### Winnie's Story: Back to Life

*By her daughter, Carol Schmidt*

*Winnie Schmidt proved that at any age, a woman can transform her health with the right attitude, the right diet and willingness to let natural remedies do their work.*

*In late 2007, at age 87, Winnie had a cancerous growth removed from her leg. The leg became infected and Winnie was given a sulfa-based antibiotic. A month later, when it appeared the infection had returned, she was given three antibiotics, including the one she had been given 30 days earlier. Soon she developed a rash, swelling in her joints and third-degree burns on her legs, arms and back. The burns, caused by an allergic reaction to the antibiotics, covered more than 60 percent of her body. Her body swelled by 50 pounds as it retained fluid due to the burns. Winnie's doctors prescribed steroids and antihistamines to deal with the allergic reaction. When there was no change in her condition, the doctors were at a loss as to how to treat Winnie.*

Chalyce Macoskey knew Winnie and her husband Edward through their involvement in a local recreation center. Chalyce researched Winnie's symptoms and realized she had developed Stevens-Johnson Syndrome, a life-threatening reaction to sulfa-based medicines and over-the-counter drugs. Winnie's primary care physician, Dr. Julia Atkins, agreed with Chalyce's assessment, as did Winnie's allergist. With the full support of Winnie's doctors, Chalyce set out to help Winnie heal by working with natural remedies. This path was the only option left for this beloved wife, mother and grandmother.

Winnie changed her diet completely, starting with substituting fresh, organic whole foods for her previous diet of fast food and pre-packaged meals. Chalyce advised Winnie in using essential oil-infused supplements and protein drinks. Chalyce discovered that organic coconut oil spread on Winnie's burns covered with sterile bandages could provide a layer of protection against infection. Essential oils for the skin, such as geranium, lavender and melrose were used to heal the burns and regenerate the skin.

With the help of these natural remedies, Winnie spent the winter recovering at home. By spring, she was healed enough to travel and re-integrate herself into a new-normal way of life, sharing her story about how at any age, quality of life can improve.

While many of those diagnosed with Stevens-Johnson Syndrome suffer devastating effects, such as lost eyesight, damage to internal organs and death due to infection, Winnie not only survived but thrived. Her doctors and hematologist monitored her progress and were amazed by her complete recovery.

As Winnie Schmidt celebrated her 91st birthday in September 2011, she continued to inspire people of all ages who were challenged with health issues. She was living proof that a combination of holistic protocols, including homeopathy, acupuncture and essential oil products can assist the body in healing itself.

What many elderly consider impossible, Winnie accomplished

daily: She shopped, cooked, walked cross country on snowshoes, and traveled to new places, all activities that she had virtually given up on because of her allergic reaction. She was deeply engaged in her life and enjoyed her "second stage of youth."

Winnie proved there can be hope in an otherwise hopeless situation when a person, with the right resources, empowers her own health and life.

Note from Chalyce: On April 29, 2013, dear Winnie earned her angel wings at 11:11 a.m. Her transition was very peaceful. We had a wonderful celebration of her life with the dear friends she had found during her second stage of life—people who were touched by her bright shining soul and beautiful blue eyes.

During the celebration of Winnie's life, as we stood on Copper Mountain, and the family spread Winnie's and her husband's ashes, two butterflies appeared and the sky turned to rainbows. With clouds shaped like angels, we felt Winnie was near and was happy! We cried and we laughed. It's a memory I hold dear to my heart.

I spent many long days with Miss Winnie and her family. I was pushed to my limits to learn, understand and coach her and her family to improve her quality of life. I prayed a lot for answers to guide this beautiful soul back to health. Because of Miss Winnie's strong will and determination, many lives have been saved. Winnie was the beginning of my creating the New Approach.

While coaching Winnie and her family, Chalyce sent this message to Dr. Bruce Fife, a certified nutritionist and naturopathic physician who wrote *The Coconut Oil Miracle* and serves as the director of the Coconut Research Center:

Dear Dr. Fife,

About eight years ago, I coached an 87-year-old client with Stevens-Johnson Syndrome. As I'm sure you know, aged people have a difficult time surviving this illness. My background is in *the use of essential oils and the use of holistic health methods to promote healing and overall health. She had burns over most of her body. Her skin started peeling, and I was at a loss. I prayed a lot and then one day I went to Whole Foods to run an errand. As I was walking and praying for something to help me save Miss Winnie, I saw your book The Coconut Oil Miracle. I grabbed it and, as if miraculously, it opened to the page about skin. I said, "Thank you, Lord!" Below the book was a shelf of coconut oil, so I dumped all of it into my cart. I raced to Walgreens to pick up sterile bandages and went straight to her home. I ran in the house shouting, "I have the answer!"*

*What saved Miss Winnie's skin was us "buttering" the bandages with coconut oil, and after we had applied the oils, we wrapped her in bandages. We did this three to four times a day for several months. Everything became about coconut oil. So, in a sense, you helped to save Miss Winnie's life.*

The meat, juice, milk and oil of coconuts have provided critical nourishment to people all over the world for generations. Coconut is a staple food for many and also provides many health benefits. Coconut oil possesses healing properties and is extensively used in traditional medicine among Asian and Pacific populations. Pacific Islanders consider coconut oil to be the cure for all illness. The coconut tree is referred to as the Tree of Life. (You can read more about coconut water and oil in the Appendix on page 146.) Only recently has modern medical science unlocked the secrets to coconut's amazing healing powers.

Here are some suggested brands of coconut water:

- CocoHydro powder (individual packets are easy to travel with)

- Harvest Bay

- Amy and Brian

- Harmless Harvest

## SHARED EXPERIENCES

### Kristine's Story: From the Couch to the Kitchen; from Tube Feeds to Real Food

*Prior to finding the Facebook group, Healing Gastroparesis Naturally, I was suffering a great deal. Four years ago, I was diagnosed with gastroparesis. The doctors just gave me pills, handed me a GP diet booklet and sent me out the door.*

*Not long after, a really bad episode sent me to three ERs before I was admitted to the hospital for four days. I wasn't given many options besides a j-tube. I refused, and spent the next few years struggling with my weight and eating. My condition got worse and worse. I eliminated more foods and beverages until I had no choice but to have a g-tube placed about seven months ago.*

*I gained weight, but was not tolerating the prescription formula and was still very ill. I had horrible stomach cramping, bloating, nausea and vomiting, explosive diarrhea, dehydration, malnutrition, insomnia, anxiety, depression and many other things. I took many different medications and was prescribed fentanyl patches. I was living on less than 1,000 calories a day and barely any fluids. I went to my local hospital each week for IV fluids. Eventually, I needed a permanent port. I was no longer taking anything in by mouth but crackers and Gatorade. Even lifting my body off the couch became challenging. Next up I was due to have my g-tube changed to a j-tube.*

*My son also suffered from horrible stomach-aches and began refusing to eat. I was so sick I couldn't even care for him. I did all I could to make it through each day myself. I can't explain how much this hurt me inside. In addition, my husband had ongoing* digestive issues from a gallbladder removal.

I was desperate, so I finally looked into the Healing Gastroparesis Naturally group I had joined on Facebook. Natural and alternative ideas were the only routes I had yet to explore. After one day of reading others' stories and all about essential oils, I ordered a GP kit. I didn't have much to lose. I checked in with my doctor and requested a month to try this "all natural" approach. I told him I was going off my medications and would start a homemade formula for my g-tube.

Three days later, my essential oils arrived. It was not a very easy start. I was extremely sick from dehydration and malnutrition and had a cold. I was also weaning off some medications that were not helping me. I was so weak my husband applied my oils the first few days every half hour. I switched from prescription feeding formula to a homemade organic formula, and started adding in kefir milk, coconut milk, chicken bone broth, coconut water and powdered goat milk. These changes allowed me to skip my nighttime pump feedings. I applied Baby's Happy Tummy essential oil on my children and started giving my family kefir milk daily. I told myself to give it a year and then evaluate the situation; after all, I was healing more than 30 years of damage.

Within days of just these few changes I noticed a huge difference. My energy, nausea, vomiting, stomach cramping, bowel movements and the amount I was feeding were all improving. I was tolerating the homemade formula, so I steadily increased my feeds. My bowel movements had changed from constant diarrhea after every feed to being normal.

After about a week following the New Approach I was getting an appetite and feeling my stomach move. A few times I even tried eating by mouth. I was feeding every two hours from early morning to night and was warming my blends to reduce stomach cramping. I was now mostly sleeping at night. Vomiting was much better except for some morning episodes. I also started becoming more active. I was extremely happy with my progress. It was not easy, but I stuck with applying my oils and pushing my feeds. Each day, I increased my formula and fluids.

Within about three weeks, I was pumping all my necessary fluids and most of my daily calories. This was a first in several years. I was doing so well I had trouble keeping up with my feeds!

A little over a month into the New Approach, I was no longer sleeping well because my body was so hungry and formula was no longer holding me over. I was shocked by how much I was getting in and that I was ready to start adding more solid foods by mouth. I went from pumping 5 ounces total fluid a couple of times a day to 14 ounces total fluid with multiple feeds a day. Before, when I was sick, I would drop down to feeding nothing at all. I never thought my nausea could be controlled, having dealt with it daily for so long. The oils worked fast to help control any nausea. I still had bad days, but they were far better than the "good" days a month before.

The kefir milk did wonders for my family. My son stopped complaining of tummy aches, and my husband's stomach and bowel movements drastically improved, too.

I continued eliminating medications, and switched from homemade formula to real pureed meals. After being on night feeds for eight months, my body was finally adjusting to not feeding at night. Eventually, I began taking in small amounts of food by mouth, a huge step from having very little oral intake.

The progress has been amazing. I'm not sure how we can ever thank Chalyce for giving us our lives back as a family. To be able to help the kids get ready for school instead of yelling orders from my bed, being able to take them to school, go to a sporting event or just tuck them in, makes every bit of this worth it! I didn't need to wait a year to know it was working.

*After two months on the program, I was able to enjoy two meals by mouth with my family on Easter. Everything I take by mouth seems to settle fine as long as I stick to clean eating and applying oils regularly. I recently added moringa leaf powder for added vitamins and nutrients. I'm always busy cleaning, running errands or making healthy food. I love doing things for my family again. Bloating and fullness have improved, and I only get reflux on rare occasions.*

*These are complicated illnesses that require a lot of attention and care. I now share with others the knowledge Chalyce shared with me. We believe in paying it forward, and have started producing kefir milk for other families where someone is suffering from stomach issues. It's helped a lot of people and that couldn't make us happier.*

*Am I perfect? No. I have good days and bad days, but my quality of life is so much better! When I went back to see my doctor he was also impressed. He told me whatever I am doing, don't stop!*

## <u>AFFIRMATION</u>

*"I no longer struggle, I simply adjust and move forward."*

–4–
# The Power of Yoga, Breath and Relaxation

*"Yoga teaches us how to breathe deeply and fully. Breathing this way brings the natural functions of the organs into balance, especially the eliminatory organs. The diaphragm and lungs expand and contract, thus massaging the internal organs... postures using the complete three-part breath can strengthen the abdominal wall and the digestive organs, supporting health and vitality.*

*In terms of gastrointestinal health, yoga allows relaxation, balancing the physiological effects of stress. Reduction in skeletal muscle tension decreases sympathetic system stimulation and subjective tension, and may improve gut motility."*
–Dr. Gerard Mullin, *Integrative Gastroenterology*

*Yoga was something I always thought of as a fad, the hippie-dippy kind of stuff where people say Namaste and Om and repeat silly chants that make no sense. I thought "Yeah, yeah, whatever, that's not for me."*

*Over the years, I tried different yoga classes to make sure I was not missing something, and though I felt somewhat better* and relaxed after a class, it never anchored me enough to keep me coming back. I was raised in the church and given the basic foundations of religion but it did not ground me in the way it does for some. Still, I've always had a feeling that there had to be something more, something to call my soul home.

In 2011, I met Dr. Lynn Crocker at an alternative medical conference in Scottsdale, Arizona. There was an immediate connection, and before I knew it, the following month I was flying back to a charity event, meeting with her and other doctors interested in aromatherapy.

Dr. Lynn picked me up at the airport and casually said she was going to yoga later and asked if I would like to join. "Sure," I said, "I'll check it out."

Wow! Was I in for a surprise! Most people in the class wore white, and their heads were wrapped in turbans. Instead of Namaste, they were chanting Sat Nam. It just went downhill for me from there. The teacher was tall with a booming presence and to be honest, I was a little frightened of it all. Dr. Lynn was smiling and beaming like she had just landed in heaven.

For the next hour and a half, I worked hard to hold the poses, stretch and balance as best I could. I heard sounds and chants that were terrifying. I prayed the entire time for help to get through the class. The teacher, Sevak Singh Khalsa, kept repeating, "Keep up and you will be kept up." I was thinking, "If I keep up I am going to die!"

You see, what we were doing that night was Kundalini yoga, which focuses on the brain and, 11 years before, I had been involved in a car accident that caused traumatic brain injury (TBI). So not only did I struggle with this yoga class being so strange on its own, but it was pushing my brain to its outer limits, and giving me challenges with my motor skills that left me flopping like a fish out of water.

*Finally, Sevak told the class, "Relax, stretch out, cover yourself up, while we do a gong meditation." I thought, "What the heck is that?" At this point, I was exhausted and my brain was fried. I collapsed and said to myself, "Okay Chalyce, here we go."*

*That gong meditation was one of the worst experiences of my life. The vibration of this percussion was overwhelming, making my head pound and my brain hurt. The yoga teacher later shared that having experienced TBI would explain why my brain felt like it was imploding and exploding all at once. I prayed for the sound to stop. It hurt my head so badly and I thought I was truly going to lose my mind.*

*When the sound finally stopped, my entire body was shaking, and I could hardly stand. Dr. Lynn bounced up, beaming from ear to ear, grabbed me and dragged me up to the teacher. I couldn't talk or think straight, and my body was still shaking. Dr. Lynn introduced me to Sevak. I will never forget this moment: He took my hand, and a sense of peace came over me. He explained that my central nervous system was "all jacked up, my friend" and Lynn confirmed how right he was by sharing that I had a traumatic brain injury. I laughed, embarrassed because he had noticed my "fish flopping," but I also realized he could see my struggle, that it was real.*

*When you have a traumatic brain injury, it is hard for people to believe you, because you may look OK on the outside. It's similar to the invisible chronic illness so many of you deal with. While Sevak held my hand, I felt a calmness I had not experienced in the many years since my accident. I shared with him that I felt like death, but I wanted to learn more. They both laughed and Sevek said, "Yes, everyone says that in the beginning. Welcome to Kundalini yoga!"*

*For the next five years, I continued to practice Kundalini yoga. I could not keep up, but I also refused to give up. Through the practice, my whole life changed; my thoughts, my world, my brain.*

*I now have tools to support me when challenges arise. But let me share this, Kundalini yoga is not for the faint of heart; it is indeed designed to help you dump your baggage and let go of the past. It brings up a lot of emotions and memories. I share with my clients to stay with it, go through the process, "let go and let God," as they say in class. I now know what this means.*

Chalyce, with encouragement and support from Dr. Lynn and Sevak, has found that practicing yoga has been critical to healing her brain and spirit. It has taken her five years to get to the point where she can start training to be a level one teacher. Although it can be quite difficult when the practice includes meditations that challenge the brain, Chalyce perseveres, because it allows her to feel clear-minded, like she felt before the accident.

The breathing, stretching and chanting of Kundalini yoga all help to heal the body on so many levels we can't even begin to understand. It is most important when you have health challenges to find that peace and balance for the brain to heal. To heal the mind, body and spirit so we can shine bright, just as we were all born to do!

## The "Wandering" Nerve and How It Relates to Digestion

The vagus nerve is the 10th and longest of the 12 cranial nerves, extending from the brainstem to the abdomen. It is involved in the parasympathetic nervous system (PNS) which controls the relaxation response, not to mention regulating the heart, lungs, upper digestive tract and other organs of the chest and abdomen.

The term "vagus" means "wanderer." The nerve is named appropriately because it wanders throughout the organs of the throat, chest and abdomen as a direct wire to the brain, in addition to the spinal nerves that also serve these body parts. The vagus nerve is principally involved with parasympathetic activity, which is largely involuntary and often emotional. It regulates heartbeat, is involved with the release of tears in crying, controls digestion and peristalsis of the esophagus and intestines, production of many hormones such as insulin, control of sphincter muscles, ovarian and uterine function, prostate function, and sexual responsiveness. It is the parasympathetic system that functions during healing and is mainly involved with protection, conservation and restoration of body resources and functions.

The vagus nerve originates from four areas of the brain and exits through the vagal ganglion at the center of the base of the skull in the vicinity of the Locus Coeruleus. The vagus nerve has 13 branches that go to all the vital organs of the body including the esophagus, larynx, lungs, heart, stomach, liver, large and small intestines, spleen and kidneys. It is through the vagus nerve that the vital functions can still be maintained even in quadriplegic people paralyzed from the neck down.

The neurotransmitter acetylcholine, released from the vagus nerve, is responsible for learning and memory. This chemical is also calming, and is used by the nerve to send messages of peace and relaxation throughout the body. In the study, *The Cholinergic Anti-Inflammatory Pathway*, research found that acetylcholine is a major brake on inflammation in the body. In other words, stimulating your vagus nerve sends acetylcholine throughout your body, not only relaxing you, but also turning down the fires of inflammation that can be related to the negative effects of stress. The inflammatory reflex may play a role in almost every disease from cardiovascular conditions to rheumatoid arthritis.

Digestive disorders can cause inflammation of the body, in time creating more and more health challenges. With that comes stress and when we are stressed we cannot relax; when we do not relax, our overall well-being is affected.

What can we do to improve quality of life and break this cycle? We can support it by stimulating the vagus nerve with breathing techniques, essential oils, chanting or singing, soothing music, meditation and conscious relaxation.

How do essential oils play a part in supporting the vagus nerve? According to *Science Daily's* article, "Could Rosemary Scent Boost Brain Performance?" researchers found rosemary oil to contain half a dozen compounds known to prevent the breakdown of acetylcholine. Students have also reported feeling livelier and more receptive to information after smelling the oil.

If rosemary essential oil can halt the breakdown of acetylcholine in the body, then when the vagus nerve is stimulated, it can transmit the proper amount of acetylcholine to the parts of the body where it is needed. Inflammation may decrease, and relaxation could become easier to obtain.

To take advantage of the benefits of aromatherapy, you may try adding your favorite essential oil to the bottoms of your feet or inhaling before doing the relaxation techniques below. Some suggested oils include lavender, Kathy's Sleep Easy blend, any citrus oil and Relax and Release essential oil blend.

## Conscious Relaxation Techniques

Relaxation techniques are a great way to help with stress management. Relaxation isn't just about peace of mind or enjoying a hobby. Relaxation is a process that decreases the effects of stress on your mind and body. Relaxation techniques can help you cope with everyday stress and with the stress related to various health problems.

When faced with numerous responsibilities and tasks or the demands of illness, relaxation techniques may take a back seat in your life. But that means you might miss out on the health benefits of relaxation.

Practicing relaxation techniques can reduce stress symptoms by:

- Slowing your heart rate
- Lowering blood pressure
- Slowing your breathing rate
- Increasing blood flow to major muscles
- Reducing muscle tension and chronic pain
- Improving concentration
- Reducing anger and frustration
- Boosting confidence to handle problems

Whether your stress is spiraling out of control or you already have it tamed, you can benefit from learning relaxation techniques. These techniques are also often free or low cost, pose little risk, are easy to learn and can be done just about anywhere. Explore techniques like those listed below and get started on de-stressing your life and improving your health.

**Kundalini Yoga.** Chalyce found the practice of Kundalini yoga worked best for her because she wanted something that could help build strength in both body and mind while keeping both moving. She is not one to sit down and meditate quietly for long periods of time.

Yoga is to yoke, or to balance us. We believe its purpose is to balance mind, body and spirit. The benefits that come along with this are toning and strengthening from the inside out while supporting the body as a whole and helping to balance the brain.

Chalyce will joke that "All other yoga was created because they could not hang with Kundalini yoga. To me it is yoga on steroids!" Kundalini combines many practices and puts them together as one, based on science, practice and research. The chanting helps focus and clear the mind. The mudra (or symbolic hand gestures) support the chanting and help move energy, making those who practice it stronger. Kundalini energy is what is created within as energy is moved up the body through the chakras (energy centers within the body that help regulate processes), bringing balance.

Chalyce believes Kundalini is the most powerful yoga one can practice.

In Kundalini, if you have fear, there is a mantra (a powerful sound, vibration or simply an intention) for it. If you need balance, there is a kriya (an exercise or group of exercises designed with an intention to move toward a specific outcome) that can be practiced. You can learn to create a practice based on what you need to improve quality of life and let your light shine.

To learn more, you can visit www.3ho.org/kundalini-yoga. Poses to support digestion that are shared in the Level 1 teaching training manual can be found at http://bit.ly/2m1eVZQ.

**Autogenic Relaxation.** Autogenic means something that comes from within you. In this relaxation technique, you use both visual imagery and body awareness to reduce stress. You repeat words or suggestions in your mind to relax and reduce muscle tension. For example, you may imagine a peaceful setting and then focus on controlled, relaxing breathing, slowing your heart rate or feeling different physical sensations, such as relaxing each arm or leg one by one.

**Progressive Muscle Relaxation.** Using this relaxation technique, you focus on slowly tensing and then relaxing each muscle group. This helps you discern the difference between muscle tension and relaxation. You become more aware of physical sensations. One method of progressive muscle relaxation is to start by tensing and relaxing the muscles in your toes and progressively working your way up to your neck and head. You can also start with your head and neck and work down to your toes. Tense your muscles for at least five seconds and then relax for 30 seconds, then repeat.

**Mindfulness Sleep Induction Technique.** This technique is designed to help you fall asleep. Begin with abdominal breathing. Place one hand on your chest and the other on your abdomen.

When you take a deep breath, the hand on the abdomen should rise higher than the one on the chest. This ensures that the diaphragm is expanding, pulling air into the base of the lungs. (Once you have this mastered, you don't have to use your hands).

- Take a slow deep breath in through your nose for a count of three or four and exhale slowly through your mouth for a count of six or eight. (Exhalation should be twice as long as your inhalation.) This diaphragmatic breathing stimulates the vagus nerve which increases the relaxation response.

- Allow your thoughts to focus on your counting or the breath itself as the air gently enters and leaves your nose and mouth.

- If your mind wanders, gently bring your attention back to your breath.

- Repeat the cycle for a total of eight breaths.

- After eight breaths, change your body position and repeat another eight breaths.

It is rare that you will complete four cycles of breathing and body position changes before falling asleep.

**Conscious Breathing.** To use this type of relaxing, diaphragmatic breathing:

- Place your hand on your low belly and allow the belly to expand and contract perpendicular to your body.

- Extend your exhales longer than your inhales. (For example, breathe in for a count of three and breathe out for a count of six.)

- Another technique is "square breathing," a simple relaxation breathing technique that can help calm thoughts and release tension. In this technique, you inhale, hold, exhale, hold, then repeat. (For example, breathe in to the count of four, hold to the count of four, breathe out to the count of four, then hold to the count of four before repeating.)

**Sa Ta Na Ma Meditation for Stress and Anxiety.** This meditation is a simple way to balance your day. It is used in Veterans Administration hospitals for patients with post-traumatic stress disorder (PTSD) and traumatic brain injury (TBI).

It can be used for everything from breaking habits to achieving emotional balance. It helps you focus and center yourself. It is a catalyst for change because it is a very powerful spiritual cleanser. You may go through a lot when practicing this meditation because you will be releasing a lot. Be present to what you are experiencing and be willing to let it all go. The process will allow you to give all your garbage back to God. If you want to maintain the status quo, don't do this meditation. If you are willing to change and welcome a new dimension of being into your life, this meditation is for you.

This meditation quiets the mind, takes away fear and builds courage to face the day. Try to practice this meditation for three minutes every day. We can all find three minutes, right?

While doing the meditation, you may experience pictures of the past come up as if there is a movie screen in your mind. Let them dance in front of your eyes and release them with the mantra. This is part of the process. If emotions come up, you can also incorporate them in the chanting. For example, if you feel anger then chant out the anger. Whatever you experience is okay. Do not try to avoid or control your experiences. Simply be with what is going on and allow yourself to go through it.

You can apply Relax and Release blend essential oil to your feet or inhale it to help you relax during this meditation.

You may try this for one minute, repeating up to 10 times. Just listening to this meditation while using Relax and Release blend may help you learn it. (You can find examples on YouTube.)

Give it a try; you have nothing to lose but your fear!

Begin your session by sitting cross-legged on the floor or seated upright in a straight-backed chair. Rest your hands on your knees with palms facing upwards. While chanting, alternately press the thumb with each of the four fingers. Press hard enough to keep yourself awake and aware of the pressure. Keep repeating in a stable rhythm and keep the hand motion going throughout the whole meditation.

1. Chant the syllables Sa, Ta, Na, Ma, lengthening the end of each sound as you repeat them with "aaaaaaaaah."
2. Touch the index fingertip of each hand to the tip of the thumb as you chant Sa (aaaaah).
3. Touch the middle fingertip to the tip of the thumb as you chant Ta (aaaaah).
4. Touch the ring fingertip to the tip of the thumb as you chant Na (aaaaah).
5. Touch the pinky fingertip to the tip of the thumb as you chant Ma (aaaaah).

Repeat 5 to 10 minutes out loud, with a whisper or in silence.

The four Sanskrit chanting sounds used in this meditation (Sa Ta Na Ma) translate to birth, life, death, rebirth.

- The first, known as the Jupiter finger (Sa), brings in knowledge, expands our field of possibilities and releases us from limitations.

- The middle, known as the Saturn finger (Ta), gives us patience, wisdom and purity.

- The ring, known as the Sun finger (Na), gives us vitality and aliveness.

- The pinky, known as the Mercury finger (Ma), aids clear communication.

We all say we want to change, or at least we want things to be different in our lives. We want to be happier and at peace within ourselves. We want more satisfying relationships. We want to be healthier. We want more meaningful work and to be more prosperous. We want to break destructive habits and stop indulging in certain addictive behaviors. The question is how can we affect these changes in our lives?

Yoga recognizes that if we want to make changes in our lives, we have to change ourselves. Yoga operates on the principle that our inner reality creates our outer reality. We have to alter our vibrational frequency so that we attract at a different level. Our frequency has to match what we want to manifest. And equally important, we have to clear our subconscious programming, so it does not sabotage our conscious intent. In fact, it is the programming in our subconscious mind that creates our reality.

According to the 3HO Foundation, "The radiance of the psyche is dependent upon the active functioning of both the pituitary and pineal glands. The pituitary gland regulates the entire glandular system. The secretion of the pineal gland creates a pulsating radiance that activates the pituitary gland. The mind goes out of balance when the pineal gland is dormant. This imbalance makes it seem impossible to break mental and physical addictions. The mantra Sa Ta Na Ma is a powerful tool to recreate balance in the mind."

Relaxation takes practice. As you learn these relaxation techniques, you will become more aware of muscle tension and the other physical sensations that come along with stress. Once you know what the stress response feels like, you can make a conscious effort to practice a relaxation technique the moment you start to feel any symptoms. This immediate response can help to prevent stress from spiraling out of control.

Remember that learning relaxation techniques is a skill. And, as with any skill, your ability to relax improves with practice. Be patient with yourself—don't let your effort to practice relaxation become yet another stressor. If one technique doesn't work for you, try another. If none of your efforts at stress reduction seems to work, talk to your doctor about other options.

Also, bear in mind that some people, especially those with serious psychological issues and a history of abuse, may experience feelings of emotional discomfort during some relaxation techniques. Although this is rare, if you experience emotional discomfort during relaxation techniques, stop what you're doing and consider talking to your healthcare professional or mental health provider.

## SHARED EXPERIENCES

### Jessie's Story: Calming the Storm

*by Chrissy Harrison*

*She was a field hockey player, local spelling bee champion and an honor student, when my daughter Jessie's life took a sudden turn.*

She began to have stomach pain and couldn't eat. Always a healthy eater, she suddenly couldn't even tolerate sips of water. We visited multiple doctors: We were told she had acid reflux, we were asked if she had an eating disorder, and we were also told she needed behavioral therapy. Sound familiar?

After an unsuccessful attempt at an ultrasound, Jessie fell into severe dehydration. As a mother, I was frustrated with the medical community. I knew my daughter, but we were being treated as if the problem was all in our heads. Blood work was normal, and she appeared normal even after losing almost 20 pounds in one month. We couldn't find an answer.

One night as I looked at my child laying on the floor (because it was more comfortable for her), I knew I had to do something. Waiting was no longer an option. We took her to the nearest emergency room. I watched as my daughter was fed fluids through an IV and given morphine. She began to smile, and I felt relieved that there must be something going on if the pain meds were working.

Five minutes later, stricken with nausea and severe pain, the morphine wasn't enough. They stabilized Jessie and moved her to a room. I was then notified that I had 30 minutes to get my stuff and make a three-hour drive to Johns Hopkins Hospital. My daughter was loaded into an ambulance headed to Baltimore. I drove behind never taking my eyes off that ambulance while tears rolled down my cheeks. At the emergency room, they began to run tests and ultrasounds. I was asked if anything happened at her birth. Was she anorexic? Suddenly, I began to question everything I had ever done as a parent. Was this my fault? What could I have done differently?

Jessie was transported to the oncology floor. They assured me that my daughter didn't have cancer, but I was never told what she did have. I tried to put on a brave face for my scared child *while trying to cope with the fact that she might have cancer. After an endoscopy and colonoscopy, they discovered inflammation and a biopsy revealed she had had a stomach virus.*

*A stomach virus? With three kids, stomach viruses were a common thing. How could my daughter be so sick without having vomited? The virus was gone from her body but left trace evidence that it was recently there. In my sleep-deprived state, I tried to remember which child had been sick and when. In fact, a week or so before she became very ill, a stomach virus had affected all three children, but Jessie had the lightest symptoms and seemed to recover quickly. Why would a stomach virus cause so many problems two weeks after the symptoms went away?*

*After an upper GI scan, she was diagnosed with gastroparesis. I thought, at least there is a diagnosis, which means there must be a cure! I had no idea I was going to spend every waking hour for the next 17 months researching medical papers, reading blog posts, watching YouTube videos…anything that mentioned the word "gastroparesis." We spent endless hours driving and seeing doctors who treated her like she was faking it or wrote her off as emotional if she cried.*

*My heart ached. I was supposed to protect her. I was supposed to have the answers. I cried a lot and felt like a failure. I wanted to give up. She wanted to give up. We were miserable. She had to leave the school she loved. She could no longer play hockey, see her friends or even eat sitting up. I prayed for an answer. Why was this happening to such a brilliant child? Would she ever have her life back?*

*Jessie was put on a feeding tube through her nose and given a little pump that would administer nutrition. We were sent home and advised to follow up in three months with the doctor. Initially, I thought she would be on it for two weeks and then be as good as new. I was so wrong.*

*She would have to fight to find a new path. She was depressed, and it was no wonder. One night, as I talked to my boyfriend, something just clicked with us about starting with protein to get her to eat again. I talked with Jessie about needing to be brave and take that step forward. She told me she was sick of being sick. The next day, Jessie took out her feeding tube. She was ready. I was exhilarated but terrified. My only comfort was the fact that my daughter found enough strength to take a step forward.*

*We started with organic scrambled eggs, apple juice and saltines. I followed the GP guidelines for low-fiber and low-fat foods, no red meat, no red sauce and absolutely no dairy or even Lactaid. Her stomach began to make sounds, and I knew we were on the right path. The excitement of having hunger pains was overwhelming.*

*Jessie began seeing a therapist to deal with the trauma of what she had gone through and continued to face. Her psychiatrist also had GP, and I felt that finally, eight months after diagnosis, we could see the light. The therapist recommended a medication to help with the tightness in her stomach. It helped but it certainly was no cure. Jessie began to tolerate more food and we kept her on a strict schedule. It seemed to help to eat at the same time every day and get plenty of rest.*

*Jessie decided she wanted to go back to school, but when school began, her body couldn't keep up with the demands. I watched a video of a girl who overcame GP with the help of a chiropractor. I found a natural healing chiropractor and things started to change. The chiropractor discovered that Jessie had a form of scoliosis that had happened seven or eight years before. She remembered falling in kindergarten on her back from the monkey bars. Jessie's curve in her back was connected to the nerves directly connected to her stomach.*

*I explained to the chiropractor what GP was and the office rec-ommended a digestive enzyme and easily digestible vitamins. After a few months of going two times a week, her back and symptoms* of GP started to improve. She had also grown and gained weight. The chiropractor recommended essential oils for digestion. All of these approaches worked, but not all of the time.

I joined a Facebook support group out of desperation. I found many people recommending essential oils from Essential7. I immediately ordered everything Essential7 had on gastro issues. Four days into using Miss Kate's Happy Tummy and Digestive 1 on a regular basis, Jessie's pain was manageable. We also used Gastro essential oil.

The combination of proper nutrition (good quality food), chiropractic care, consistency and most importantly, essential oils from Essential7, have given her a better quality of life in the last 17 months than she had on any prescription. We began seeing a traditional Chinese medicine (TCM) doctor who explained the correlation between the spleen and heart. Jessie is currently on TCM herbs and doing much better.

Healing is a process that takes time. You have to stick to the plan. You cannot eat food that causes inflammation and expect the essential oils to fight through it. It all starts with the right nutrition. Meditation and relaxation techniques calm the mind and help calm the nerves connected with the stomach. Yes, we should all be able to eat a pizza when we want. Maybe someday Jessie will. I wouldn't have that kind of hope without these little bottles of oil that have calmed the storm inside my daughter's stomach.

## AFFIRMATION

*"I cast off the burden of fear and doubt so I can go free, happy and harmonious."*

## –5–
# Putting It All Together: Trying the New Approach

*"What lies behind you and what lies in front of you,
pales in comparison to what lies inside of you."*
–Ralph Waldo Emerson

## SHARED EXPERIENCES

### Stephanie's Story: Learning How to Eat Again

*During some of my most rock-bottom moments (or perhaps days, weeks, even months) I would find myself drowning in hopelessness from the diagnosis of an incurable disorder, so scared of the pain that at times it felt as though I was paralyzed with fear. Over the years, I have come to recognize the terrible downward spiral these feelings can lead to, as the body's response is to freeze. It makes sense if you consider what happens in fight or flight, with freeze being an additional, often common reaction, especially for those living with PTSD.*

*Not only did I physically and mentally feel worse, my body began to slowly shut down. I'm sure some of you can relate to this vicious cycle. When loved ones told me to relax I got angry and when doctors brought up an eating disorder I wanted to explode. How can they not understand the pain, nausea and feeling like a bowling ball was sitting in my stomach? Those were the reasons I didn't want to eat. Even when forcing myself at times, I would just end up doubled over, unable to handle sitting up for another bite.*

*So I understand that when our New Approach addresses learning to eat it may seem impossible or overwhelming. Learning a new reality may feel like more than you can handle when you are suffering so much. After all, isn't being sick hard enough? Who wants to face the crippling fear of how a food or beverage might cause the body to react?*

*About two years ago, when I was drowning in this fear, a couple of close friends helped me. They understood how hard I had tried but also saw how restricted and isolated I had become. Not only with food but with all aspects of life. In the beginning, the push to "try harder" hurt and I didn't want to listen. How could they possibly understand what I was going through?*

*But eventually I saw it, too; I had to get my life back. The change took time. I started with baby steps like spending just one hour a week volunteering, reading to kids at an elementary school, where a friend would drop me off and pick me up. I learned that if I could breathe through it and somehow learn to observe the pain, be one with it, as opposed to fighting and fearing it, then slowly I could gain control of the pain or discomfort.*

*One of these dear friends shared the quote below with me. The writer, Kinsey Jackson, battled with her own chronic illness. She was diagnosed with a number of autoimmune diseases in her 20s and was forced to make some difficult changes in her life. She is now a clinical nutritionist and writer for the web site Paleo Plan, where she writes about the benefits of real food and the importance of having the faith, courage and persistence it takes to give our bodies the best opportu-*

*nity to reclaim health and vitality. No matter what your beliefs may be, we can all practice having this faith; the trust that we are strong enough to persevere. Easier said than done of course, but in my experience, absolutely life-saving at times.*

*"Fear and faith are two sides of the same coin, in my opinion," Kinsey Jackson writes. "The more you have of one, the less you have of the other... they are inversely proportionate. I think that ultimate faith requires us letting go of needing to understand 'why' or 'how.' Trust that God knows 'why' and that through our living and breathing we will become the 'how.'"*

Why talk so much about fear and emotions under the topic of how to eat again? For our bodies to have the absolute best opportunity to digest food, they must not perceive food as a threat. Fear prepares us to react to danger. Once we sense fear, our body releases hormones that slow or shut down functions not needed for survival and sharpen functions that might help us survive. Oxygen moves away from our digestive tract and flows into our limbs. Our heart rate increases and blood flows to specific muscles so we can run faster. Hormones flood an area of the brain known as the amygdala to help us focus on the presenting danger and store it in our memory.

So, understanding this cycle of pain = fear = more pain, what can we do to stop it? The following excerpt from a Huffington Post article written by Peter Abaci, M.D., "A Radical Shift to Better Pain Relief," explains it nicely:

"Nerve cells in the brain have the ability to change their function and structure based on both external and internal factors. These changes can ultimately shape the way a person thinks and feels. Chronic pain, on the other hand, is the disease. It is a complex equation of physical, emotional, cognitive, genetic and environmental factors that come together with the end result that leaves us hurting in some way, day after day. It is in the chronic pain setting that the neural plastic properties of the brain can lead to maladaptive changes in the brain's wiring that both make us feel lousy and change our behaviors into seemingly a different person. True healing requires re-wiring these adverse changes into something more positive and less taxing to the brain. Unfortunately, many of the typical treatments offered for pain problems—like painkillers, injections and spine surgeries—offer little chance of reversing the chronic pain brain. But stimulate the brain to change, and the potential to reverse the course of a person's chronic pain experience can become an effective treatment strategy."

In other chapters, we have gone over some proven strategies of meditation and relaxation to change the "pain brain." Here a few additional quick tips on moving past fear and learning to eat again:

- Recognize fear while believing in the process.

- Pay attention to the small markers of progress along the way and celebrate them.

- Read through the stories shared in this book from others who were extremely challenged and able to bring their bodies and life back in balance.

- Remember to take things slowly—as some days, especially in the beginning, may be more difficult.

- Seek support from friends, family, online groups, etc.

- Ask for help in preparing foods and having them ready in portions you can start with.

- Take time to breathe deeply before eating to help relax the digestive tract and mind.

- Trust the ideas and tips shared throughout this book are going to support you during your journey.

Choose organic food whenever you can or at least be mindful of the pesticides, herbicides and hormones found in foods. Additives, preservatives and artificial ingredients in foods today may contribute to the constant inflammation we are challenged with. Shop local when possible and talk with farmers when you can. Many of them are very mindful in their farming practices, but simply cannot afford to be certified as organic. If you're buying seafood, go with wild-caught, not farm-raised. There are also great resources online and, in addition to natural markets, Sam's Club, Walmart, Target and Costco now offer cleaner choices to appeal to more mindful customers.

Next, we offer steps in a regimen that has helped people begin to heal their digestive challenges. You may find it helpful to keep track of what supports you over time. Your journal is a great place to keep a running list as a reminder of what you *can* do!

## Try the New Approach

Taking small steps will start you on a healing path. Here is a list of steps previous clients have followed. These ideas combine foods, essential oils and mindful practices in a way that has been effective, even for clients who have not eaten solid foods in a long time. We suggest you follow these steps as best you can, always paying attention to what your body can best tolerate.

- First thing each morning, you may start by applying oils to the bottoms of your feet before getting out of bed. Suggested oils include Gastro, Kate's Happy Tummy and Turmeric.

- You may try drinking 1 teaspoon of Himalayan salt sole

(see chapter 9) in 5 ounces of water, or if that is not supportive to you, 1 teaspoon of sauerkraut juice may be substituted for the sole. Raw apple cider vinegar is another alternative, depending on what your body tolerates best.

- It is suggested to wait about 20 minutes after the sole, kraut juice or raw apple cider vinegar before having any kefir or yogurt. Taking the two together may create a challenge.

- Take the kefir out of the refrigerator so it can warm to room temperature. You may add blueberries, raspberries or strawberries to it when you feel able to incorporate them. If you are unable to try kefir, the Bulgarian yogurt suggested in chapter 3 is an option. White Mountain or Stonyfield Organic whole fat are two yogurt brands we suggest. Start with 1 to 2 ounces.

- You may try adding ¼ to ½ teaspoon of moringa powder to the kefir or yogurt. Once quality of life improves, we suggest using moringa powder every other day and then as desired, but not to be taken daily long-term. According to WebMD and Organic India, the brand suggested and enjoyed most by clients, "Moringa is a nutritionally complex superfood naturally abundant in vitamins, minerals and amino acids—the building blocks of protein. Moringa is considered one of the most complete, nutrient-dense plants on earth and an important food source in some parts of the world. Because it can be grown cheaply and easily, and the leaves retain lots of vitamins and minerals when dried, moringa is used in India and Africa in feeding programs to fight malnutrition."

- Breakfast can be anything that sounds good and that is

supportive to you. Some examples are: a scrambled egg in a small amount of coconut oil or butter with cooked baby greens such as spinach, bok choy or kale; cheese (when tolerated); kitchari; hot cereal such as rice, quinoa, oatmeal or cream of buckwheat; toast with nut butter; smoked salmon; chicken or miso soup; or even some leftover dinner from the previous night. Some of these foods may sound unconventional, but previous clients with GP have been able to try them in small bites.

- Portion size is key and something to be mindful of with digestive challenges. Some of Chalyce's clients wait a half hour after eating a few bites of breakfast to see how they are feeling and then try a couple more bites, continuing this process until quality of life improves. You are in control of how and what you eat. Always do what works for you, and in time, your body will respond positively.

- If solids are a challenge, you may try sipping clean (meaning antibiotic-, hormone- and steroid-free) chicken broth or bone broth, which is very supportive to the body. If you are unable to cook, most grocery stores now carry organic broths that you may heat up, being mindful of ingredients. Keep in mind microwaves are not ideal to warm foods, as they can deplete some of the nutrients that are vital to supporting the body.

- Another liquid option is to experiment with protein powders. If you know you can tolerate a smoothie, you can add a small amount to one or, as Chalyce often suggests and has had success with, try protein powder in a little kefir or Greek yogurt (organic or hormone- and steroid-free).

Suggestions include Organic Plant Protein by Garden of Life, Warrior Blend Raw Vegan Protein by SunWarrior, Great Lakes or Vital Proteins Collagen protein, and Plant Fusion Phood, an organic plant protein with added fermented foods. Remember to try in small amounts, 1 to 2 teaspoons to start, or half the normal serving.

- Remember, Gastro and Kate's Happy Tummy essential oil blends before eating may help with digestion. Apply 4 or 5 drops on the bottoms of your feet or simply inhale.

- We suggest trying to eat every two hours to support and rebuild the body until you feel that you can eat small meals. Do what is best for you. This is only a suggestion.

- Set a reminder alarm so you do not go too long without eating.

- If you are out, you may carry snacks with you. Suggestions include Amazing Grass bars, GoMacro bars (many clients have done well with these, but always be mindful of what and how much you tolerate), crackers, cheese, nut butter, clean deli turkey and Orgain protein drinks. The best snacks are supportive of improving quality of life; not foods that deplete the body, forcing it to work harder, like highly processed and fast foods.

- Remember to eat small amounts when necessary so the stomach is not overwhelmed, triggering the challenges you might have encountered before.

- It is suggested to wait 15 to 20 minutes after drinking before having anything to eat. Try to limit liquids with your meals and wait about 15 minutes after eating before having a drink, as liquids can dilute gastric juices and digestive enzymes. Research in the study of Ayurvedic medicine has shown that these restrictions may be beneficial in reducing challenges with reflux.

- Try to avoid cold foods and drink. In traditional Chinese medicine, it is suggested that liquids and food be room temperature because cold foods may slow digestion.

- Staying hydrated is key. Drinking room temperature coconut water may help with hydration and electrolytes as does adding a small amount, just one or two small crystals of Himalayan sea salt to your water.

- You may try sipping on Yogi Stomach Ease tea once a day to help with digestion. Note, this tea may have a laxative effect, so drink it in small amounts to support digestion. Previous clients have found 2 to 3 ounces a couple of times a day to be helpful.

- Remember that stress can bring on bouts of diarrhea, constipation or nausea. These challenges are not always the GP acting up, but may be the body reacting to conditions. If you experience these challenges, work on making it a practice to regroup, drink some kefir or whatever you find most beneficial (such as Stomach Ease tea), breathe deep, practice the meditation Sa Ta Na Ma (see page 61) 10 times, apply Relax and Release oil and move forward.

- Essential oil tips:

  ° You may try Relax and Release oil blend when you are

getting anxious or feeling uneasy. You may apply 4 or 5 drops on the bottoms of your feet or simply inhale.

○ You may try the Quease Go Away essential oil blend when you are challenged. You may apply 4 or 5 drops on each foot or inhale until quality of life improves.

○ You may try turmeric essential oil for gas, bloating or upset from being full. You may try applying 4 or 5 drops mixed with 15 drops of carrier oil, on the bottoms of your feet, or simply inhaling.

• During the day, be mindful of your fruit intake. Others have found they do better with high-glycemic fruits after 3 p.m. eaten by themselves, while low-glycemic fruits, such as berries, are okay through the day if they can be tolerated.

• We suggest being mindful of heavy protein intake after 3 p.m., as some have found this may increase the unpleasantness associated with stomach challenges. Proteins that have worked well for clients include fish, a little chicken or turkey, crackers, cheese, soup, yogurt, butter or cultured cheese with crackers, smoked salmon, well-cooked split mung beans (see ideas for kitchari in chapter 9), sprouted and cooked quinoa, cooked veggies and basmati rice. After your challenge of upset stomach has passed, you will find you may eat whatever clean proteins you like in small portions.

• After 7 p.m., it is suggested to limit heavy snacks or late eating if possible, as this allows the stomach to rest and heal rather than focus on digestion. If you feel out of balance and can't go long periods of time without eating, you may try the following suggestions:

- ° Sheep or goat cheese and crackers (gluten-free if possible, or organic, corn-free) are good for evening snacks, or some cooked apple.

- ° When tolerated, try uncooked apple (remove skin) with some nut butter, cultured yogurt or kefir. With Chalyce's clients she has found that when starting the New Approach, a bite or two of apple with almond butter worked well and helped to provide satiety at night as well as support blood sugars. Remember, this is a process! Once the stomach is balanced and you are comfortable, you may try gradually increasing the portion size.

- ° If you wake up hungry in the night, you may try the following: your favorite healthy gluten-free or sprouted bread toasted with nut butter; a few bites of Amazing Grass bar; cheese or nut butter and crackers.

The goal of these daily practices is to begin to see improvement in your quality of life. It is important to remember you will have good days and days that are still not as good. If you have a day that is more challenging than usual, go back to the basics until you feel back in balance. Keep in mind healing is a process: Be patient and eventually it will come together for you.

Often, progress depends on education and effort; the more effort you put into achieving balance, the better the results. No one can do that for you, it is up to you and you only. We can provide the tools, but to improve your quality of life, you have to put those tools into practice. During this lifestyle change, you may want to refer to the above suggestions as a gentle reminder to keep your hopes high and moving forward.

---

**JOURNAL EXERCISE: TRACKING WHAT WORKS**

To improve quality of life, write down how the day is going so you know what foods may trigger your particular challenges and which oils seem to support you most. This record of your triggering foods and helpful practices will become a very important reference for you.

1. Did I start my day with Gastro, Kate's Happy Tummy and turmeric oils?
2. Was I mindful not to eat too much at one time?
3. After I ate, how did I feel? How about later in the day?
4. What are my go-to essential oils that seem to improve my quality of life?
5. Is my nausea caused by being hungry?
6. When did I last eat?
7. Am I eating heavy foods late at night?
8. The changes are subtle, am I paying attention and writing down the positives?
9. Did I overeat or combine foods that made me feel uncomfortable?
10. What are the oils I use when I feel uncomfortable?
11. Did I practice Sa Ta Na Ma when I was feeling upset or anxious?
12. Could any medications I'm taking be creating more challenges? Do my doctors know and can I set up a time to discuss this with them?
13. Are there foods I can eat that are easier to digest?
14. Am I noticing that each day I am getting better?

---

## AFFIRMATION

*"I am doing the best I can."*

# – 6 –
## Do Our Emotions Contribute to Disease?

*"The greatest mistake in the treatment of disease is
that there are physicians for the body and physicians
for the soul, although the two cannot be separated."*
–Plato

Modern science confirms what most of us may already know: Negative emotions can contribute to illness. In the My Body + Soul article "The Five Emotions that Make You Sick," we found this quote that may help you better understand why the emotional connection is important.

"The neurotransmitters that fire in the brain connect with our hormones, immune cells and organs, contributing to disease and poor health. Likewise, the precise nature of the disease itself cannot be linked to a particular emotion. For example, a previous condition such as pneumonia or a severe fall could predispose you to lung infections or back problems. In addition, conditions such as asthma, arthritis, heart disease and diabetes may include a genetic factor. However, a stressful event may just be the straw that breaks the camel's back, and the trigger for that disease to surface, after lying dormant for years."

Now before you begin to worry too much about worrying, the news is not all bad. Just as negative emotions can create disease, positive emotions and uplifting thoughts can also help create better health.

You know that feeling you get when something exciting is about to happen? Maybe your heart flutters or you suddenly feel a jolt of energy? How about when you feel scared or anxious? Goosebumps, nausea or difficulty breathing may occur. This is your body responding to emotions. Exactly when and where one may become ill as a result of negative emotions cannot be accurately charted. The extent of the damage of an emotion or stressful event (think those with post-traumatic stress disorder) may take years to develop into a condition such as cancer, or may erupt immediately in an attack of shingles or an outbreak of cold sores.

So can our emotions actually make us sick?

As Lissa Rankin, author of *Mind Over Medicine: Scientific Proof That You Can Heal Yourself*, shares, "With all those negative emotions filling her mind and all those stress hormones coursing through her body, no vegetable, supplement, exercise program or drug was going to be strong enough to counteract the harmful health effects of chronic stress responses on her body."

How common is it that a doctor, or perhaps one of the many specialists we often end up seeing, will make the statement, "it's all in your head" or "have you tried working with a therapist or taking anti-depressants?" But we feel the pain; we know it is real! Bear in mind that there is solid science behind the connection to our emotional experience and illness. Now don't give up on us yet, we truly believe what you are feeling is real!

We believe, and so research has shown, that illness can

begin with our emotions. Chinese medicine has held on to this theory for thousands of years, that illness can be rooted in our emotions. Traditional Chinese medicine also strongly believes, as we do, that healing the mind may also heal the body. It is a challenge to change your thoughts, especially when weighed down by a serious health condition. Through practicing mindfulness every day, Chalyce has worked hard to break habits ingrained for more than 40 years. Is it worth the work, the hope that we can feel better, even when we may be told it's not possible? Yes!

We can choose to be mindful of ourselves and not be victims, blaming people for the way we feel, for what happens to us or why we are the way we are. Blaming no longer serves us. We have to own up to our own actions, feelings and current state. We can choose to make our best effort to be healthy, happy and whole. Emotions are part of being human, and they will continue to be a part of us whether we like it or not. The best course of action is to acknowledge when you are experiencing an emotion without beating yourself up about it.

The word affirmation comes from the Latin *affirmare,* originally meaning "to make steady, strengthen." Most of us don't realize how powerful our words are, whether spoken out loud or in our daily thoughts. When you're feeling angst, try repeating positive affirmations to yourself to help rewrite those negative emotions. Say them to yourself at least 10 times a day. Other options include writing an affirmation into your journal each day, sharing affirmations with family and friends to repeat back to you as reminders, or using sticky notes to post them in areas you see frequently, such as your bathroom mirror, nightstand, car door, office desk or doors around the house. You may use the ones we suggest at the end of each chapter as examples and decide what works best for you.

# Suggestions for Experiencing Specific Emotions

According to *Chinese Medicine Living*, "Emotions are of course a natural part of being human. Feeling joy, sadness and anger are all perfectly normal experiences we have in our day-to-day lives. It is when these emotions become excessive or are repressed and turned inward, that they can become pathological and cause disease."

Here are five emotions that may contribute to illness according to traditional Chinese medicine (TCM), the affected organ, as well as suggestions for correcting them from the website My Body + Soul (www.bodyandsoul.com.au). In addition to the suggestions from that site listed below, we have added which essential oils may be beneficial for each emotion.

## Resentment

Traditional Chinese medicine (TCM) practitioners believe resentment affects the liver and gallbladder.

You may sip lemon juice and honey in hot water each morning, golden milk (see recipe on page 117) or your favorite tea such as chai or green tea. You may use the essential oil blend Relax and Release to let go of resentment. Gently inhale, or you may apply 3 or 4 drops on the bottoms of each foot or 1 or 2 drops on the wrist as desired.

**Affirmations:**

"I am willing to release the past."

"I choose to look for positive attributes in each person."

**Activity**: Anything that may get your mind off stewing and fuming. Examples may include: volunteer work, creative writing, sharing with and supporting others can all be beneficial when we tend to focus on negative thoughts.

## Worry and Overthinking

According to TCM, worrying and overthinking can affect the spleen, tampering with food digestion and nutrient absorption.

You may try to avoid caffeine and sugar. Enjoy soups, stews and warming foods. Things that comfort and calm the mind and spirit.

You may try the essential oil blend Courage, gently inhale or apply 1 or 2 drops on the wrist or 3 or 4 drops on each foot as desired.

**Affirmations:**

"All will be well."

"I am calm and safe."

**Activity**: If you can, try petting a purring cat or snuggle with a dog. In her book, *Animal Assisted Therapy in Counseling*, professor of counseling and director of the Consortium for Animal Assisted Therapy at the University of North Texas, Cynthia Chandler reviewed several research studies on the psychophysiological and psychosocial benefits of positive social interaction with a pet, such as holding or stroking an animal. Benefits include: calming and relaxing, lowering anxiety, alleviating loneliness, enhancing social engagement and interaction, normalizing heart rate and blood pressure, reducing pain, reducing stress, reducing depression and increasing pleasure.

Breathing into your belly or doing the meditation Sa Ta Na Ma (instructions on page 61) can be very beneficial. Listen to your favorite music or go for a walk in nature.

Worry is a common affliction. We worry about money, career, exams, loved ones, not to mention our health challenges. While it is important to ponder life's problems, worrying will not help. Remind yourself of this and find a practice that works for you.

## Guilt

According to TCM, guilt and shame are associated with the bladder.

Allow yourself one "guilty pleasure" a day that won't negatively impact your health. For example, take a long nap, treat yourself to a massage, plan a date night or jump on the bed!

You may try Happiness essential oil blend to lighten your heart and enjoy the day. You may apply 1 or 2 drops on the wrist or 3 or 4 drops on each foot as desired or gently inhale.

**Affirmations:**

"I am doing the best I can."

"I release the need to blame myself."

**Activity**: Find yourself a grassy patch, lie in the sunshine, cuddle under your favorite blanket or soak in the tub. Know this is what you deserve and don't even think about doing anything else.

## Grief and Sadness

Both of these emotions can affect the lungs according to TCM. Golden Milk (see recipe on page 117) is a lovely way to comfort the soul.

Mountain Spirit Blend may be a great way to support you when you have been overcome with grief. You may try 1 or 2 drops on the wrist, 3 or 4 drops on bottoms of feet or gently inhale when desired.

**Affirmations:**

"I will be gentle with myself as I recover from my loss."

"My heart will heal."

**Activity**: Join a choir or sing in the comfort of your home. The vibration of singing helps release stored pain. Even the sound of music can be soothing and ease challenges with grieving.

Whether from the death of someone close, the loss of a relationship, or perhaps facing the possibility of a career or life dream that may not come true, grieving is part and parcel of being human. Seek support and give yourself compassionate time to heal.

## Irritability and Anger

This emotion is associated with the liver according to TCM.

A soothing cup of tea of your choice is beneficial because of our sense of smell and taste.

You may try Relax and Release blend to help let go of resentment. Gently inhale, or you may apply 3 or 4 drops on the bottoms of each foot or 1 or 2 drops on the wrist as desired. Any essential oil that you find pleasing can create the shift you are looking for.

**Affirmations:**

"I seek peace and harmony in myself and for all those in my life."

**Activity**: Try learning to meditate. Meditation will be an excellent skill for you, helping to increase the buffer zone, allowing things and people not to get under your skin. Again, referring to Sa Ta Na Ma meditation on page 61 is very beneficial. A walk outside for a few minutes can also bring you back to a more positive place.

If you would like to dive a little deeper into this subject, try reading *The Biology of Belief* by Bruce H. Lipton, Ph.D. According to reviewer Dr. Wayne Dyer, the book "is a groundbreaking work in the field of new biology and it will forever change how you think about thinking. Through the research of Dr. Lipton and other leading-edge scientists, stunning new discoveries have been made about the interaction between the mind and body and the processes by which cells receive information. It explains how genes and DNA do not control our biology, but instead, DNA is controlled by signals from outside the cell, including the energetic messages emanating from our thoughts. Using simple language, illustrations, humor and everyday examples, he demonstrates how the new science of Epigenetics is revolutionizing our understanding of the link between mind and matter and the profound effects it has on our personal lives and the collective life of our species."

Another helpful resource is Dr. Dyer's book, *Excuses Begone! How to Change Lifelong, Self-Defeating Thinking Habits*. In it, he proposes asking yourself seven questions that may help you shift your beliefs:

- Is it true?

- Where did the excuses come from? What's the payoff?

- What would my life look like if I couldn't use these excuses? Can I create a rational reason to change?

- Can I access universal cooperation in shedding old habits?

- How can I continuously reinforce this new way of being?

The things we tell ourselves when seeking that balance between body and mind can have a huge impact on how we feel and the goals we hope to reach. Those goals may be different for each of you. Maybe it's taking pain down on the scale from a 10 to a 3, having more energy to be with your family, the ability to try a new food, or sleeping peacefully through the night.

An audio version of *Excuses Begone!* is also available on YouTube for free. Chalyce listens to it before bed and in the morning to create that shift she is seeking. It is very powerful and she has found it can be life-changing for those she has worked with.

When we are sick and struggling every single day with our health, it is easy (and completely understandable), to get frustrated, to want to give up hope some days. Of course we want to get better, of course we want to get out of bed, take part in activities, be there for others. There are days that will be hard, but, with this New Approach, our clients now enjoy good days, and when those days come, it is important not to fall into old habits.

Start by making a small change in your vocabulary by removing the word "but."

*Examples:*

"I do feel a little better BUT how long will it last?"

"I am open to the New Approach, BUT it requires me to focus and think and I don't have the energy to do it."

With a chronic and traumatizing illness like GP, it is easy to succumb to the victim mentality. Instead, we should believe that we really do control the outcome of what happens to us. Our words and thoughts are powerful; and when we let go of excuses, as Dr. Dyer explains, then it makes room for the positive. This, in turn, can create a shift and even though things may not be perfect, we feel better because of that shift. Our surroundings don't change, but how we begin to perceive them does.

## Self-Talk Shift

Chalyce recalls how a friend started her on a helpful path:

*I asked a good friend and student once, "Why do I have to struggle and run into roadblocks every time I get back on track? Something or someone always stands in my way. I am good, honest, thoughtful, caring, but still, horrible things continue to happen."*

*The student asked who the common denominator was in each of the challenges I described. I thought about it... Oh my gosh, it was me! I was in the middle of this downward spiral.*

*He reminded me that no matter what terrible things may happen to us, how we choose to react to those things predicts the outcome. I could decide to take control of my life and my emotions, instead of playing the victim over and over.*

*Seven months have gone by since this awareness occurred and I have been creating an environment where I am no longer a victim of my circumstance. I do see a shift; subtle changes that are bringing positive things to my life through this change in thinking. Is it easy? Absolutely not! Painful? Absolutely!*

*Listening to and reading Dr. Dyer's book and hearing from other experts has shown me that, yes, while I am human, I am in charge of what happens to me, or at least how I choose to take on what happens. As painful as it is, I can change. I can change my health, my mind and my spirit.*

## Healing the Spirit

As part of our healing, we have to understand that there truly is a mind-body-spirit connection, and if we fail to create balance with all of them, then part of us may not heal as it should. Now, we don't mean that you have to go to church or join some new-age community that is going to enlighten you. We are suggesting that you find something that connects you to the universe, God, spirit, Mother Nature--whatever you believe in and connect to--you have to find it, and when you do you will create that shift of peace that allows more healing within yourself.

Illness begins at the level of the spirit. Disharmony or disease of the body can often be the result of disharmony or disease in the spirit. When we address the spirit, when we work to heal our emotional well-being, we often experience fewer physical manifestations of disease and illness. We have been on this journey most of our lives, searching for some balance and peace within but not knowing how to get there. We have also been where you are, living with health challenges. What we have finally begun to realize is that if we can learn to control our emotions, then we have a better chance of taking control of our health.

Many things affect our emotions: pregnancy, childbirth, diet, lack of exercise, illness, death or even stress. The emotions around memories of powerful events in our lives are especially potent in unsettling our peace of mind. Unfortunately, when this onslaught of emotions attacks, we often seek medical attention in hopes of easing our distress. But medicine is often a temporary fix, the treating of symptoms instead of treating the actual cause of distress. Sometimes the temporary fix can lead to even more challenges than before.

Emotions are an addiction. Every time you revisit the emotional drama of a memory, you reinforce that emotion and make it even stronger. How can you neutralize negative emotions? Try this: To help break negative emotions, bring up a memory. Think about how the emotions around that memory make you feel. Does the emotion and the feeling own you? Does it control you?

Ask yourself, does this emotion have the right to own and control me? No? Then let it go! As you release the emotion, letting it go, affirm that the emotion does not own or control you. As you make this affirmation, apply an essential oil as suggested below. In time, you will notice the grip of the emotion easing, until ultimately, it will no longer have a hold on you. Although the memory will remain, the emotional drama no longer controls you.

## Emotions and Essential Oils

The beauty of essential oils is that they work with the body's chemistry to help restore the balance of the mind, body and spirit. Essential oils are drawn from the vital energies of nature's many plants, making each oil or blend very diverse in its effects. Essential oils work in many different ways. The benefit of an oil depends on its chemical properties. Some individual oils can have 200 or more different properties. These various properties are why lavender oil, for example, can be used for stress, burns, rashes, bug bites and so much more.

Essential7, which produces only oils of the purest and highest grade, offers several blends created to take the guesswork out of using oils to enhance emotional healing and harmony. These oils may be used topically, by diffusing or inhaling. An experienced practitioner who is knowledgeable about the use of essential oils will understand the ideal oil blend, delivery method and body placement to address specific imbalances for each individual.

Here are some essential oil blends we suggest:

- **Courage**: This brave blend may be useful for occasions when you know you will be outside your comfort zone such as job interviews, public speaking, trying a new food, etc., as well as for an extra energetic support boost. Rub a few drops of Courage onto the soles of your feet or your wrists, or rub a few drops vigorously between the palms of your hands, then cup them around your nose and breathe deeply.

- **Enlighten**: For use with yoga and meditation. This blend may help some to reach a state of higher consciousness.

- **Relax and Release**: May be used to help relieve stress and stress-related conditions. Aids in yoga and meditation.

### Meditation and Chanting Exercise for Dealing with Emotions

Find a place in your home that you can set up as your special meditation place. This can be a corner of a room or a comfortable chair. If it can be in a bedroom or some private place, that is even better. Your meditation area does not have to be fancy, but if you have room to create a "healing place," please do so. You may put flowers or a picture of significant meaning in this space. You can also simply hang a picture on the wall in your meditation corner to help remind you this is a place for you to become quiet and turn your eyes inward to your own beautiful self. Every time you meditate in this place, you will be setting the energies for powerful healing to occur at all levels of your life. The energies will naturally build over time the more you sit there in contemplation. Meditating, chanting or repeating positive affirmations are some of the best things you can do, as any change we attempt immediately brings up anxiety. Eliminating and reducing anxiety is the very first step to improving quality of life.

Instructions for meditation:

Turn off your cell phone. Make sure you will not be disturbed. You may try the Relax and Release oil blend for this meditation. Sit in your meditation place and get comfortable. Use pillows if necessary.

Close your eyes. Take a long deep breath. Exhale. Take another deep breath and exhale through the mouth and let go of your day. Open a bottle of a suggested essential oil such as Relax and Release and either put a drop on your hand or simply breathe in deeply from the bottle. If you put a drop of essential oil in the palm of your hand, circle it three times to open up the aroma and the essence of the plants. Circle the oil with awareness, thinking of how the plant grew on this planet, and the earth has given this gift to help you. Allow gratitude to begin to rise in your heart. Breathe the essence of the oil in through your nose deeply, breathing up through the nose and above the head into light.

Exhale and allow yourself to begin to let go. Breathe in again deeply, 500 feet above your head into beautiful, loving light. Exhale, letting the light begin to sprinkle down in and around your body, washing any heaviness out of your body, as though you are in a rain shower of light.

Breathe in deeply again, looking up into the light, hold your breath a moment, connect to the light, turn the breath outward and exhale through the mouth, allowing any heaviness to leave your body, like blowing smoke out of the mouth.

Continue to take long, deep breaths. In through the nose, up into the light and out the mouth, until you can breathe light into your body, and exhale light out the pores of your skin. Sit quietly. Observe the sensations in your body. Allow radiance to shine out of you into the room. Absorb this beautiful energy.

Gently open your eyes. Send gratitude and approval to yourself. Put your hands on your heart and breathe in and then out of the heart, for a few additional minutes.

## SHARED EXPERIENCES

### Courtney's Story: The Difference a Month Can Make

*I want to give everyone something to think about that may give some hope, instead of always hearing stories of discouragement. I have cystic fibrosis (CF), which I have found many times allowed me and my health concerns to be taken seriously by doctors.*

*I was admitted to the hospital in October 2014, after losing about 12 pounds over a month's period, and vomiting 10 to 15 times a day for the previous six months. During my stay in the hospital, I was given IV pain medication and had a feeding tube inserted. After six weeks, I went home, still on pain medication. After asking both the acute and chronic pain team to get me off these meds, I was refused and sent home on them. When we went back to the hospital a month later for a follow-up, I again asked for help getting off the narcotics, and again was refused.*

*Before this hospital stay, I took some Tylenol for pain only when needed: not daily. It was not until I was recently hospitalized for a severe bowel obstruction, that I found a doctor who agreed to help me and my family, along with a psychiatrist who specializes in pain* management and practices at the same hospital I had been admitted to. By the end of the stay, I was told I was on the equivalent of 1,000 mg of morphine per day. I'm 5-foot-2 and weigh 110 pounds. Nearly every nurse who heard about my heavy morphine dose was shocked.

With the doctor and psychiatrist's help, I was taken off the pain medication and only had about an hour of very few withdrawal symptoms. I was put on something different, and haven't looked back. My entire life has changed since coming off the pain medications. I have had almost no pain, compared to daily severe, excruciating abdominal pain. My diet is very strict, I follow what Chalyce and others from the Healing Gastroparesis Naturally Facebook group have suggested. The difference I feel in myself is indescribable; the difference others see, is even more. For anyone feeling helpless and in pain and thinking this is the end of your life—you should know that if it worked for me, it can work for you, too! You just have to be willing to change your lifestyle. I had been sick for years before finally getting help.

The psychiatrist who took me off the pain medication told me that it is normal to feel good for a few months, but then some pain can come back. He said the best thing you can do for this is as much research on mindfulness as possible and try to connect the body with the brain. I've taken one course in mindfulness already, with a few more lined up.

I know I'll have good days and bad, but the difference in my life today versus a month or two ago is night and day. I feel amazing, and I wish the best for the rest of you as well.

## AFFIRMATION

"I choose to be happy, healthy, whole and bless who and what I am, whatever that means for me at this moment."

# –7–
## Our Children's Challenges

*"The moment you doubt whether you can fly,*
*you cease for ever to be able to do it."*
–J.M. Barrie, *Peter Pan*

It seems today there are more babies, children and teenagers experiencing more and more health challenges. To start with, we believe food is our biggest obstacle. Our fast-paced lifestyle, which leaves little time to prepare home-cooked meals, not to mention time to sit down and eat them together as a family, has made way for fast and highly processed foods to become the norm. This does not effectively support and sustain a healthy body. It fills a void in our stomachs, and perhaps our minds temporarily, but does nothing to nourish our bodies. The nutritional value of these processed foods is very low or non-existent.

Second, research continues to show how the overuse of antibiotics is creating challenges with our digestive system, interrupting healthy flora in the intestines. Healthy intestinal flora supports our immune system; therefore, an imbalance of gut bacteria equals a weak immune system. In turn, lots of children become sick, and it becomes a cycle that never ends. When antibiotics are overused, inflammation sets in, creating, in our opinion, lifelong chronic health challenges.

And to top this off, many of today's conventional foods contain GMOs (genetically modified organisms) and chemicals. If growers spray fruits and vegetables to kill bugs, fungus and bacteria, plus feed their animals food laden with hormones, steroids and antibiotics, what is this going to do to us when we eat those fruits, vegetables or meats?

Agricultural herbicides and pesticides affect the digestion in the insects that eat them. What does it affect when we ingest those substances? If they feed hormones and steroids to animals to fatten them up, grow quickly, and yield more meat and milk, what is meat from those animals doing to us and our children? The article, "Three Reasons Your Daughter's Puberty Won't Be Like Yours," that ran in *Time* on January 9, 2015, highlighted the work of researchers Louise Greenspan and Julianna Deardorff, authors of *The New Puberty*. They decisively pointed to three major risk factors responsible for this difference; obesity, chemicals and stress. "Most of the chemicals in common use today were developed after World War II, the same time we began to observe a rise in the onset of early puberty," they write. The authors suggested steering clear of chemicals, including antibiotics found in meat and dairy, which can act like hormones once in a child's system.

If you are challenged in the area of digestion, then your children may have the same challenges. If the quality of food does not improve, and digestion is not supported, then their quality of life will be compromised as well. Below are suggestions shared by the mothers in our Healing Gastroparesis Naturally group, including essential oil blends made specifically for children.

## Essential Oils for Children

Baby's Happy Tummy blend was originally created for a child named Brooklyn, based on specific information about Brooklyn's health challenges her mother shared. Other parents in the Healing Gastroparesis Naturally group found it helpful for babies to receive 1 or 2 drops of the oil blend on the bottoms of feet and for toddlers to receive 2 to 3 drops. For children 6 to 12 years old, 4 or 5 drops on each foot every hour when challenged is suggested, or before meals. Parents will also sometimes use a diffuser, or add oils to cotton balls, and place them on air vents in the home or car to help calm and improve the quality of life.

A good resource for the whole family is *Aromatherapy for the Healthy Child,* by Valerie Ann Worwood. This book is easy for beginners and may be used for both children and adults. Be sure to check out the videos where we share instructions for the use of oils in children under the age of 6 and children ages 6 to 12. (Go to www.essential7.com for a link to the videos.)

## Digestive Support

Supporting healthy intestinal flora is imperative for our children. You can find kefir in many flavors that children find appealing. It is lactose-free and, as always, the best choice would be organic and from grass-fed sources if possible. A teaspoon on an empty stomach is suggested two to three times a day if possible to start, and then over time you may increase to 1 to 2 ounces a day. Children find kefir very soothing to the tummy. The Latta USA brand would be our first choice, if you live in the eastern part of the United States. The brand is making its way across the country, so it may be available in other regions soon. Stonyfield Greek Yogurt includes the probiotics that we suggest, and it comes in a delicious vanilla flavor. If dairy is a challenge, some parents buy or make water kefir and add organic fruit juice, which seems to do the trick. Kristine Krebsbach, who we lovingly call the Facebook group's GP Kefir Queen, has some great tips on how to make your own kefir. She is a great lady with her own miracle story about improving the quality of life with our New Approach. (See page 48.)

When your children are challenged with eating or drinking, a suggested go-to is Orgain for Kids. This is the cleanest product we have found geared for children and includes a healthy balance of nutrients. We suggest using Orgain temporarily and not as a substitute for meals. Orgain is great when it is challenging to find something that will be supportive and begin to improve quality of life.

Amazing Grass Kidz Superfood is another beverage option that may support your children if they are challenged with upset tummies. It is available in both berry and chocolate flavors.

## Hydration

To help keep children properly hydrated, we suggest coconut water. Because coconut water can be pricey, you might consider buying it in powdered form. One source is a company called Big Tree Farms, which is mindful of people, our planet and their production process. The company's Coco Hydro and Coco Hydro Sport come in a powder form so it is more affordable and you can use less than the directions suggest, depending on your child's taste. It is very pleasant and a better choice than most sports drinks that use high-fructose corn syrup, artificial dyes and flavors that can make challenges worse.

Recharge drink is another suggestion that health food stores and some grocery stores carry, if you need something quick and cannot find Coco Hydro. It is also a better alternative than the sports drinks.

The key to a healthy child is providing nutrient-dense foods and staying away from processed, fast foods or boxed foods. The "cleaner" the better. Simple ingredients and fewer chemicals will give your child's body support in a positive way and improve the quality of life faster. There are many websites with great recipes and suggestions for feeding your children fun nutritious meals. For a list, check out the article "Top 5 Websites for Healthy and Organic Recipes for Kids" on the website Green & Clean Mom (www.greenandcleanmom.com).

And don't forget we have families on our Facebook group who will be happy to give you hope, support and great ideas so that you don't feel alone. We are here as your GP family with help to improve quality of life for the whole family.

## SHARED EXPERIENCES

### Brooklyn's Story: A Child's Journey with GP

*By her mother, Tracy Church*

*I could talk for hours about Brooklyn, but I will try to keep this short. I had a lot of problems during pregnancy which led to being seen by high-risk doctors. At the first sign that our baby was in dire trouble, she was delivered by emergency c-section. She had started shunting blood from her stomach to her brain, depriving her stomach of the oxygen and nutrients needed to function properly.*

*As a preemie, Brooklyn was not able to breastfeed, so I pumped my milk and fed her through a supplemental nursing system until she was strong enough to take a bottle. She received breast milk for several months.*

*After that first day in the hospital I noticed something wrong; she was eating, but minutes later was throwing up. The doctors said it was normal, but I fought to have her seen by a GI doctor. The first test they ran was an upper GI scan with a pH probe. Next, they did a gastric emptying study that showed she had digested only 20 percent of her food in four hours.*

*We ended up trying seven different medications. The last one worked for a short time, but when Brooklyn turned two we made the choice to discontinue all of them because of the possible risks of long-term use. She seemed to do okay off the medications, so the doctors said she had outgrown the gastroparesis.*

*About a year after stopping the meds, she started having stomach pain, nausea and occasional vomiting. I knew something wasn't right, but I got a lot of resistance; people told me I was feeding her too much, or to not let her eat fruit because it was too hard on the stomach.*

*Well, this mama has some fight in her. I took Brooklyn back to the GI to find out what was going on. She was diagnosed a second time with GP, so I started researching anything and everything that might help. I realized that going organic was the only solution. It has been several months since trying to switch to clean and organic food; we still have a way to go due to state laws forbidding buying and selling of raw milk. But we are doing our best for our little girl.*

*When she started the clean diet, Brooklyn stopped vomiting, but she still had pain, nausea and constipation. Chalyce sent us the essential oils for gastroparesis and they have been a godsend. Since starting them, Brooklyn has only had pain three times. Each time I applied the oils and her pain and discomfort disappeared within 30 minutes.*

*Now Brooklyn wakes up asking for food instead of getting out of bed only to head to the couch immediately, crying because it hurt too much to even sit up. She is finally starting to gain weight at the age of four. At her last check-up she was finally on the growth chart at 5 percent and is still on the chart now. I honestly believe if it wasn't for Chalyce and Kathleen Atkins (who also assisted in sharing ideas), and everyone else in the Healing Gastroparesis Naturally group, I would still be trying to figure all of this out on my own.*

*Two and half months since starting the New Approach, Brooklyn is no longer complaining of pain with the help of Latta Kefir, Vita Coco Kids coconut water and Baby's Happy Tummy oil. She can eat pretty much whatever she wants as long as it is clean or organic.*

*Brooklyn still has her days, mostly just with acid reflux, but we have been able to control that the best we can with apple cider vinegar. We use the oils once in the morning and once at night and some during the day if the need arises. As I am writing this, it has become a new year, and my hope for Brooklyn and all of you is for everyone to take charge and get that quality of life we all deserve.*

## AFFIRMATION

*"I am bountiful, I am blissful, I am beautiful,*
*I am the light of my soul."*

# –8–
# Managing Migraines and Hormonal Imbalance

*"If you don't like something, change it. If you
can't change it, change your attitude."*
–Maya Angelou

Many of us have experienced migraines at one time or another. The underlying cause has baffled doctors for years. We do know that one of the triggers may include food allergies. When people say they have food allergies, we immediately start thinking about digestion and elimination. In our society today so many are victims of fast food or processed foods. We know that many of the ingredients in fast food are harmful and can negatively affect the way we digest and eliminate our food. Trupti Gokani, M.D., board-certified neurologist, shared her take on migraines associated with digestion in an article featured on Huffington Post. Here are some takeaways:

"Food allergies, often considered hidden since they are not obvious to many clinically, are very commonly found in our migraine patients. Out of 500 patients tested, upwards of 60 percent had allergies to dairy, about 50 percent to grains and 35 percent to eggs. Many of these patients had *hidden* food allergies. They didn't even realize the offending food was creating an allergy response in their digestive tract since they didn't present with digestive symptoms.

"Migraine attacks involve excitable neurons that are often quieted with serotonin, a neurotransmitter believed to be mostly produced in the gut. Note, this is the neurotransmitter linked to the success of triptan medications, the largest class of FDA-approved abortive medications for a migraine. The neurons, in later stages of a migraine attack, become inflamed—translation: pain.

"The gut has its own enteric nervous system; some call it the 'second brain.' The digestive system makes serotonin at optimal levels when it is functioning well."

When we are unable to digest properly, our elimination becomes compromised. You may have bouts of constipation and/or diarrhea. Later, you may have challenges with diverticulitis, irritable bowel or inflammatory diseases such as Crohn's. At some point, our lifestyle becomes a stressor on our bodies, and our body starts talking to us by way of such disorders. These disorders can go beyond digestive challenges and may include migraines. According to the Mayo Clinic, research has shown that people who regularly experience gastrointestinal symptoms such as reflux, diarrhea, constipation and nausea, have a higher prevalence of headaches than those who don't have gastrointestinal symptoms. In many cases, childhood periodic syndromes evolve into migraines later in life. Conversely, these studies also suggest that people who get frequent headaches may be predisposed to gastrointestinal problems.

As we discussed in chapter 2, when it comes to food preparation, many herbs and spices are far more useful than just helping food taste better. They play an important part in digestion and the functioning of the pancreas, gallbladder and liver.

Looking at different nationalities, Italians cook with rosemary, thyme, oregano and basil; Chinese cook with ginger, fennel, star anise, peppercorns, cinnamon and lemongrass; East Indian cooking includes curry spices such as turmeric, coriander, cinnamon, red chili pepper and cardamom; Hispanics tend to prepare food using many spices and herbs including cumin, cilantro, chipotle, saffron, cloves and chilis. Interestingly, using the variety of food additives mentioned above can actually help us digest our foods, therefore reducing chances for additional challenges such as migraines.

You will find many of these plant derivatives in the essential oil blends suggested below, like peppermint and ginger, which you may find improve quality of life, specifically when it comes to migraines, hormonal and blood sugar challenges:

- **Gastro**: 4 to 5 drops diluted with 6 drops of a carrier oil and you may apply to the area of concern, diffuse or apply to the bottoms of the feet before eating.

- **Digestive Blend #1**: you may use as suggested above.

- **Turmeric**: 2 to 3 drops diluted with 15 drops of a carrier oil applied as suggested above.

- **Rosemary**: 2 drops diluted with 4 drops of a carrier oil and apply as suggested above.

You may always apply more if needed. Therapeutic grade essential oils are very concentrated so a little goes a long way. Remember to dilute with a carrier oil if applying to areas other than feet.

## Dehydration

Not all migraines are caused by food. Dehydration is a common contributor as well because most of us do not drink enough fluids. Studies have shown that up to 75 percent of Americans are chronically dehydrated. Coconut water is suggested as a simple fix to help hydrate the body and provide nature's electrolytes. Himalayan salt can be useful, too (more details are found in chapter 3). Keep in mind that flavored waters, energy drinks and electrolyte replacements may be filled with synthetic chemicals and high fructose corn syrup. You might as well save your money and grab a soda. Well don't do that, but you get the idea! When you need hydration, you can't beat coconut water and water with added Himalayan salt.

## Hormones

Hormones can also be another challenge and can cause individuals to suffer from migraines. Having consistent estrogen levels may improve headaches, while experiencing estrogen levels that dip or change can make headaches worse. These changes can happen to women just before getting their period. It is also important to look again at your diet. If you eat unclean meat that has steroids and hormones added, where do you think those added chemicals go? This can cause an overabundance of hormones in our system, creating havoc in our bodies.

Suggestions for handling emotional and stress-induced head-aches could include utilizing Enlighten, Courage and Relax and Release essential oil blends. You may want to try applying the oils on the base of the neck, over the heart or just by simply in-haling. Please avoid direct sunlight during outdoor activities or the use of tanning beds when using Enlighten.

## SHARED EXPERIENCES

### Stephanie's Story: Finding Balance with Clary Sage

*To say my hormones have been a mess is an understatement.*

Back in 1999 at the age of 19, I had my very first surgery for endometriosis and ovarian cysts. The doctors compared the size of these cysts to softballs. At the time, I was getting ready to start college classes, and was in a new relationship with a man who is now my loving and dedicated husband. The experience of disease and surgery was pretty traumatic. In fact, this was the very beginning of my body taking a slow roll downhill. The treatment plan included birth control pills with hopes that course of treatment would prevent the endometriosis and cysts from returning. The medication worked, but I began to experience reflux, mood swings and food sensitivities.

By 2005, as a newlywed, I was back in the hospital needing the same laparoscopic surgery. I decided to get off the birth control pill regimen and see how my body would do on its own. For the next seven years, I experienced amenorrhea, which is the abnormal absence of menstruation. Long story short, everything came back in 2013, after going through an intense two weeks of daily myofascial bodywork. However, within a year I was regretting this return to a monthly cycle: My periods were more frequent, heavy and extremely painful with the addition of migraines during this time.

Fast forward to 2016, with the suggestion from Chalyce of using clary sage essential oil, both on my lower abdomen and bottoms of feet, I finally experienced a somewhat regular cycle. An unexpected but pleasant benefit of using clary sage is that I am sleeping through the night and actually feeling tired at bedtime. Insomnia has plagued me for years, and this is the first time something has worked besides prescription medications, which can be highly addictive.

I personally relate a lot of my digestive issues to hormonal and sleep cycles so though I am still working on managing the *digestion piece, this experience only gives me hope that this New Approach we are sharing is real and can make a difference!*

## AFFIRMATION

*"Today is a better day than yesterday and tomorrow will be even better."*

# –9 –
# Recipes for Healing Gastroparesis Naturally

*"He who takes medicine and neglects to diet*
*wastes the skill of his doctors."*
- Chinese Proverb

Despite everything that has happened over the years, follow-ing a nourishing, nutrient-rich diet has played a key role in Stephanie's well-being, whether it's a cup of homemade broth and small bites of pureed foods during a flare, or on the good days, maybe some roasted veggies and baked fish. She feels lucky to be able to eat with such a serious challenge like gastropare-sis and feels grateful for the opportunity to share some delicious recipes with others who may find them just as comforting in times of need.

Combined with the other ideas provided in this book, these recipes could be a great start to a new journey, one of living your best with GP and following our New Approach. Remember to start with small portions, chew, chew, chew, and know the food is bring-ing you the goodness your body needs, one small bite at a time.

Making smart, nourishing choices when it comes to food doesn't have to be complicated. In fact, when you begin to feel the impact from the changes it is hard not to begin finding joy again in the kitchen!

It is all about taking small steps, so you will find this section includes basic ideas to get started. We have categorized the recipes into four sections:

- **Part 1** includes some of the digestive aids discussed throughout the book including Himalayan salt sole, kefir using both dairy and water grains, miso soup, golden milk and bone broth.

- **Part 2** lists recipes for easy-to-digest soups and porridges.

- **Parts 3 and 4** are short, with recipes for two veggie dishes of Moroccan sweet potatoes and roasted zucchini. Also included are two ways to prepare easy-to-digest pancakes.

Remember, when you incorporate the essential oils, meditations, digestive aids that you tolerate best and other suggestions found throughout this book, you will find that trying new foods can be a completely different experience than before, when you did not have the added support. Take it slow and experiment with what sounds good. In your journal, keep track of what works well for you, celebrating as you begin to see the small changes and, in time, are able to enjoy more and more of both food and life.

# Liquids to Assist in Digestive Support

## Himalayan Salt Sole

Water and natural salt are foods, not medicines. Due to their special properties, they give us energy and have a balancing, neutralizing and detoxifying effect on our bodies. There is no better natural means than these to stimulate the body's own regenerative capacity and restore our equilibrium. Thus, water and natural crystal salt have a positive effect throughout the body. With the help of the sole drink you have the opportunity to become or stay healthy, to rediscover your physical and emotional equilibrium (inner harmony) and to boost your energy levels.

### Supplies/Ingredients:

- Glass jar with plastic or non-metal lid

- Filtered water

- Himalayan salt crystals

### Directions:

1. Fill clean, glass jar about a ¼ full with salt crystals.

2. Top off with sufficient, good quality, low mineral-content water, to cover the crystals well. Leave about an inch of space at the top.

3. Seal the container to prevent any contamination.

The crystals will dissolve in about two hours and the concentrated sole mixture will then be ready to use. The warmer the water, the more rapidly the salt crystals dissolve.

For a sole drink, take up to a teaspoon of concentrated sole from the container, using a non-metal spoon and add to a glass of water. Stir vigorously. When the sole runs low, simply add more water. Make sure at least one crystal is always visible in your sole concentration. This is your guarantee that the sole is saturated with salt. As the level of salt sole lowers, you may add more water. When there are no more salt crystals left, add some more and wait. If they dissolve, then add more until they no longer dissolve. A saturated sole will keep indefinitely. Neither bacteria, viruses nor fungi are able to multiply in it.

## Kristine's Dairy Kefir Milk

### Supplies/Ingredients:

- Quart size glass jar
- Coffee filter
- Rubber band
- Plastic or stainless steel strainer with fine holes
- Bowl with pour spout that strainer can sit in
- 1 to 2 teaspoons milk kefir grains (live are best)
- Organic whole milk (raw is best), goat's or sheep's milk are options if better tolerated

### Directions:

Place 1 to 2 teaspoons of milk grains in the quart-size jar. After you add the grains, fill the jar with milk, leaving about 2 inches of space at the top to allow for expansion. Cover the jar with a coffee filter and a rubber band to allow the mixture to breathe.

Store in a dark place for 24 hours, then pour the milk through a strainer into a bowl, reserving the grains and jar. Fill a jar from the bowl. If tiny air pockets develop in the bottom of the jar, the strained milk is fermented and can then be stored in the fridge. If a second ferment is needed, pour the strained milk in additional jars, filling only half full, as the mix can expand and separate quite a bit. Cover with a loose lid and store in a dark place for another 24 hours.

To make more kefir, use the reserved grains and the first jar, add more fresh milk and repeat. Using the reserved grains and the unwashed jar helps start the fermentation process.

## Kristine's Water Kefir

### Supplies/Ingredients:

- 1 quart size jar

- Rubber band

- Lid for the jar (fermentation lid if you would like a more carbonated beverage)

- Bowl

- Plastic or stainless steel mesh strainer with fine holes

- 4 tablespoons water kefir grains

- Spring water

- ¼ cup raw organic sugar

- Drip of molasses

### Directions:

Add about 1 inch of warm spring water to the quart-size jar. Next add your sugar and molasses. Stir until sugar is dissolved. Fill your jar with room temperature spring water, leaving 1 to 2 inches of space at the top. Add water kefir grains to the jar, then cover with a coffee filter secured with a rubber band. Screw on lid over coffee filter, making sure it's not completely tightened. This allows gases to escape so pressure does not build up. Too much pressure and your jar may explode. If you would like a more carbonated beverage use a fermenting lid for this process.

Place water in a dark place to ferment for 24 to 48 hours. Small bubbles should rise to the top and water should have a different, more sour smell. Place strainer over a bowl and strain out the grains. Place strained kefir water in the fridge or on the counter for a second ferment. If doing a second ferment, pour in a jar and cover with a semi-tightened lid. After 24 hours, place in the fridge.

To make more water kefir, use a clean jar, add your grains and repeat the process. During the second ferment, you can add various items such as fruit or herbs to enhance the flavor. Please check online for recipes.

## Miso Soup

A fast, simple and nourishing soup.

**Ingredients:**

- 1 cup water
- ½ tablespoon miso paste

**Directions:**

Bring 1 cup of water to a boil, then add ½ tablespoon of miso paste. Reduce heat, then let simmer, without letting it boil, for 2 to 5 minutes.

**You may also add near the end of the cooking time:**

- 1 teaspoon of Moringa powder (high in iron and B vitamins)
- Cooked white rice
- Protein of choice such as a bit of cooked white fish, shrimp or shredded chicken. You can also whisk in a lightly beaten egg and simmer an additional 2 minutes.

## Golden Milk

Golden milk can be a wonderful, warm beverage to sip on in the evening. The turmeric and ginger are well-known to help aid in inflammation and digestion and pair well with the sweet creaminess of milk and honey or syrup.

**Ingredients:**

- 1 cup of milk or dairy-free milk such as unsweetened So Delicious Coconut
- 1 teaspoon dried turmeric
- ½ inch of freshly grated ginger
- Dash of black pepper (optional)
- Honey or maple syrup to taste

**Directions:**

Bring milk and spices to a low simmer in a saucepan over medium heat, being sure to stir well. Allow to heat for another minute, being careful to not let the milk overheat. Continue to stir, remove from heat, and allow to sit for about 10 minutes to improve the infusion of ingredients. Pour milk through a strainer to remove ginger, and serve warm. This is best taken in the evening before bedtime.

## Nourishing Bone Broth

Making homemade bone broth is a great routine to start. Stephanie enjoys making it on Sundays with an organic, whole chicken. This creates enough delicious broth to use in soups and porridges as well as enough to freeze for when times get busy. Every one of us is different in terms of what we can eat and drink, as well as the severity of our symptoms. If you are currently on a liquid diet, try just sipping the broth. Over time add a bit of rice, then you may try to work in some protein (blended if necessary). This broth is not difficult to make, so give it a try, even if it is just for sipping small amounts throughout the day as you start to follow the New Approach.

### Choosing Ingredients

If making broth is new to you, then the easiest way to start is by using parts leftover from a whole roasted chicken, whether home cooked or store bought. Try to use organic or pasture raised chicken when possible, and avoid any meat with added hormones and antibiotics. Use the chicken as a dinner for the family or friends, saving some of the chicken breast meat for yourself, if you can eat it.

Some stores sell bags of soup bones. If you can't find any in the grocery store, ask your local butcher or farm. Options can include a whole chicken, or as mentioned, leftover roasted chicken or turkey bones, beef knuckles, marrow bones or oxtails. Beef broth can be a little on the heavier side, so it may be best to experiment with chicken or turkey in the beginning.

For a simple version, you can just place a whole uncooked chicken in a stockpot with a few chunks of peeled and chopped carrots. Add about a teaspoon of Himalayan sea salt, bring to a boil, lower heat, cover and simmer for 3 to 4 hours. Follow step 3 below to strain, cool and store.

**Tools for Cooking:**

- **Stockpot.** This is the most traditional way of simmering stock on low for several hours.

- **Slow cooker.** May be preferred method of cooking because you can leave it alone to do its magic during the day or overnight.

- **Pressure cooker.** Extracts all of the nutrients and flavor in a short time. The Instant Pot is also great for soups, porridge and rice. The website NomNomPaleo (www.nomnompaleo.com) shares a recipe for the Instant Pot, just make sure to use our GP-friendly ingredients.

**Directions:**

1. Place 1 to 2 pounds of bones in pot and cover with cold water. Add 2 tablespoons of apple cider vinegar and let sit for 30 minutes to an hour (optional). This pulls the nutrients and minerals off the bones for a more nutrient-dense soup.

Vegetables and herbs can be added, but if you are sensitive to many foods and have a hard time with digestion, then you may choose to omit them for now. Otherwise, start with those that tend to not cause bloating and upset such as:

- 2 or 3 peeled and chopped carrots

- 1 stalk of celery chopped

- Handful of green chives

- 1 or 2 slices of fresh ginger

- 1 or 2 teaspoons of favorite dried herbs such as oregano, basil, marjoram and thyme

- Fresh parsley added during the last 10 minutes of cooking

2. Simmer on low for a minimum of 8 hours. If you are using a pressure cooker like the Instant Pot, check the instructions for cooking time. Poultry can be cooked 12 to 24 hours, while beef bones may cook longer. (Some people better tolerate a broth made with just 1 to 2 hours of cooking time, so you may choose to start there and see how your body does.)

3. Remove the bones. Next, fill sink with ice and water and place a separate pot topped with a cheesecloth-lined strainer in the ice bath. Pour the hot broth through the strainer into the pot sitting in the ice. Stir the broth until cool, then refrigerate. Once completely cooled, the fat will solidify on top of the broth, and can be scooped off and discarded. At this point, you may divide the broth into containers, saving enough for the next few days, and freeze what's left.

*Tip! Freeze broth in ice cube trays. In a standard size tray, each cube is ⅛ cup, making it easy to measure out what you need to defrost.*

# Easy-to-Digest Soups and Porridge

## Kitchari

Kitchari is a wonderful staple when you are sick, when you are feeling emotional or stressed, for your kids or a loved one when they are under the weather, and when you are low in energy and need to gain some strength. You'll be surprised how warming and comforting it is, and soon it'll be the stuff your cravings are made of. We modified the recipe so it is GP-friendly. If you can't find these ingredients at your store, you can buy packets of kitchari from Banyan Botanicals at www.banyanbotanicals.com.

Split yellow mung dahl beans are available at Asian or Indian grocery stores, health food stores or on online. Different spellings include mung or just dahl. Please note that you do not want the whole mung beans, which are green, or yellow split peas.

### Ingredients:

- 1 cup split yellow mung dahl beans (soaking up to 12 hours is best for digestive challenges)
- ¼ – ½ cup uncooked white basmati rice (you may soak up to an hour)
- 1 tablespoon of fresh ginger root, grated
- 1 teaspoon each of cumin and turmeric powder
- ½ teaspoon each of coriander and cardamom powder
- 3 cloves of garlic (optional depending on tolerance)
- 3 bay leaves
- 7 to 10 cups water or organic chicken broth
- ½ teaspoon salt (Himalayan salt is suggested)
- 1 small handful chopped fresh cilantro leaves

- Can add steamed vegetables or clean meat for extra blood sugar support.

*Tip! For weak digestion, gas or bloating, soak beans overnight and then drain. Or, before starting to prepare the kitchari, first par-boil the split mung dahl (cover with water and bring to boil), drain and rinse. Repeat two to three times. Cook as directed.*

**Directions:**

Wash split yellow mung beans and rice together until water runs clear. In a pre-heated large pot, dry roast all the spices, (except the bay leaves), on medium heat for a few minutes. This dry-roasting will enhance the flavor. Add dahl and rice and stir, coating the rice and beans with the spices. Next, add water and bay leaves, then bring to a boil. Boil for 10 minutes. Turn heat to low, cover pot and continue to cook until dahl and rice become soft (about 30 to 40 minutes). The cilantro leaves may be added just before serving. Add Himalayan salt to taste. You may also add a little coconut oil or ghee to support the digestion of vitamins and minerals.

## Congee

This simple rice soup is easily digested and assimilated. In China, it is traditionally eaten as a breakfast food where ingredients may be chosen for their specific medicinal properties. The chicken and broth, for example, build strength and are especially good for wasting illnesses (where disease can cause muscle and fat tissue to "waste" away) and injuries. The ginger and cumin boost flavor and aid in digestion, plus, each offers additional medicinal benefits.

Congee is easy to make in a crock pot. Put the soup together before going to bed and awaken to this satisfying porridge. Or, you may start in the morning and the soup will be ready when you come home for a nourishing dinner.

Note: All ingredients suggested in the recipes should be as clean as possible. Chemicals create more challenges for the digestion. It's very important to choose beef that is grass-fed and free of hormones, antibiotics or steroids. Fruits and vegetables should be pesticide-free, herbicide-free or organic. Many local farmers have organic practices but cannot afford the certification. Support local as much as possible, and ask about farming practices. It is also important that the animals are treated humanely.

**Ingredients:**

- 4 to 6 cups broth, preferably homemade: Use less for thicker porridge, more for soup consistency
- ½ cup uncooked jasmine or basmati rice
- 1 slice ginger root, organic or chemical free
- ½ teaspoon Himalayan salt
- ¼ teaspoon ground cumin
- Optional: GP-friendly vegetable(s) of your choice (chopped

carrots, sweet potato, winter squash, mushrooms, etc.) You may add what works for you, and remember, organic is preferred, but pesticide- and herbicide-free vegetables are just as good.

**Directions:**

**Slow Cooker:** Stir all ingredients in slow cooker and cook on low overnight for breakfast, or during the day for dinner. Before serving, remove ginger slice. When not tolerating food well, eat small portions of soup throughout the day. For breakfast, you can add an egg, a bit of soy sauce or coconut aminos and a teaspoon of coconut oil to the congee. You could also add more water and a bone-in chicken breast as a full meal for dinner. Or, if you have leftover chicken, turkey or white fish, they are great add-ins as well.

**Stovetop:** Use the same ingredients, then bring to simmer in saucepan. Set to low, cover and allow soup to cook for 1 to 1½ hours.

For additional information and ideas, check out Paul Pitchford's book *Healing with Whole Foods*.

## Bieler Broth

Are you looking for a way to incorporate more vegetables in your GP diet? This refreshing and light soup digests easily. It was created by Dr. Henry Bieler, author *of Food is Your Best Medicine*. The recipe has been adjusted to include the taste of celery, but not the actual blended celery. However, if tolerated, feel free to include the celery. Both zucchini and green beans are excellent sources of potassium and sodium. When prepared and cooked right, these green veggies digest surprisingly well. Add in some simmered ginger and fresh parsley, both wonderful digestive aids, and you have a nourishing soup.

Each ½ cup contains less than 2 grams of fiber and can be sipped warm or cool on its own. Enjoy added to white rice or some diced potato with optional protein such as egg, fish, tofu or chicken for a complete meal.

### Ingredients:

- 1 medium zucchini, skin peeled
- ½ cup frozen green beans
- 1 stalk celery
- 1 thin slice of ginger
- Handful of parsley leaves

### Directions:

Begin by chopping zucchini into thin slices and celery into two to three large pieces. Add to pot with ½ cup of green beans, a slice of ginger and enough water to cover veggies. Bring to a boil and cover with lid, turn down to low heat and allow to simmer for 20 to 30 minutes.

Remove celery and place into blender with parsley, adding

enough water to make about 2 cups. Blend well and enjoy immediately, or allow to cool. Broth can be refrigerated for a few days or frozen.

*Tip! Freeze in ice cube trays for future soup cubes, easy to defrost and reheat in GP-friendly portions (each cube = ⅛ cup).*

## Journey with Gastroparesis Create-A-Soup

As you well know, there is no "one size fits all" when it comes to our food choices. That is why it's best to create "you friendly" meals by combining the ingredients that work best for *you*. Soup is just about the most forgiving meal to make and there are so many ways to make it work for you. Stephanie's kick-the-cold soup is one of her favorites and most comforting food anytime. It is a basic broth-based soup with added carrots, zucchini, ginger, Herbs de Provence seasoning, sea salt and rice.

Mixing this up is so easy! If rice doesn't settle for you, simply don't use it or add some potato or sweet potato, or serve with a slice of gluten-free bread. The possibilities are endless. Here are some of the staples to begin building a great soup.

- Liquid: Meat, fish or veggie broth (preferably homemade and clean, chemical free)

- Vegetables: Choose one or two that you tolerate well: carrots, peeled zucchini, potato, sweet potato, winter squash, parsnips, pumpkin, green beans, greens (like spinach, kale or bok choy), leeks, onions, mushrooms, asparagus.

- Protein: Shredded or ground chicken or turkey breast, fish or seafood such as shrimp or cod, or an egg stirred in to the soup and cooked for 2 minutes before serving. Tolerate dairy? Add some organic milk and/or shredded cheese.

- Seasonings: Experiment with your favorite herbs or spices. Some favorites are thyme, oregano and basil; dill; turmeric and ginger; or a blend of savory herbs called Herbs de Provence.

*Tips!*

- *For a thicker, heartier soup, the addition of potatoes, white rice or pasta can be great and create more of a meal if well-tolerated.*

- *Coconut milk can also help to create a chowder-like soup.*

- *Hand mashing or pureeing are options to make soup easier to digest, just remember to sip slowly and always "chew" to stimulate the digestive enzymes that begin in the mouth.*

- *Make sure to simmer veggies until very soft and easy to break down. Harder root vegetables like carrots usually take the longest: Slice them thinly and cook 30 to 60 minutes.*

- *Add in dried herbs in the beginning and fresh herbs in the last 5 to 10 minutes of cooking. Cooked meat can be tossed in at the end or follow instructions for timing and cooking in the soup. Most meats require 5 minutes or less when cut in small pieces.*

## Sweet Potato Cream of Rice

A great way to use leftover baked sweet potatoes for a soft, easy-to-digest sweet and savory bowl of comfort. You can make your own cream of rice by placing uncooked white basmati rice into a food processor or blender and blending until it's a fine consistency and will cook in a short time. Bob's Red Mill has creamy rice that you may try as well.

**Ingredients:**

- 1¼ cup water
- ¼ cup cream of rice
- ⅛ teaspoon sea salt
- ⅛ teaspoon cumin and cinnamon or Moroccan Spice Blend (see recipe for Moroccan Sweet Potatoes)
- ⅛ cup cooked mashed organic sweet potato

**Directions:**

Bring water to a boil and slowly whisk in rice and spices. Turn heat to low stirring constantly for 1 to 2 minutes (4 to 5 if using blended rice). Remove from heat, cover and let sit for a few minutes, then add in mashed sweet potato and stir until well blended. Serve warm immediately.

**Add-in Options:**

- Replace half the water with unsweetened almond or coconut milk.
- Use homemade broth in place of water or pour some over at the end.
- Use turmeric as an added body-support spice.

- Divide into smaller portions and add a soft scrambled egg for extra protein or a small piece of chicken or fish to the side for a complete meal.

## Buckwheat Pumpkin Porridge

Pocono Organic Cream of Buckwheat cereal is an excellent way to bring a little variety into your breakfast, especially on a cool morning when nothing sounds better than a bowl of hot, tasty cereal. There are many combinations you can use, whether it is cooking with coconut or almond milk, adding pureed fruit, spices, an egg or nut butters.

**Ingredients:**

- ¼ cup cream of buckwheat
- 1 cup water
- ¼ cup coconut, almond milk or hemp milk
- ⅛ teaspoon Himalayan salt
- ⅛ teaspoon of warm spices (cinnamon, nutmeg, cardamom or the Moroccan Spice Blend)
- ⅛ cup canned pumpkin (Farmer's Market is a great organic brand)
- ½ - 1 tablespoon of peanut or almond butter, depending on what you best tolerate, make sure it's organic if possible
- Drizzle of maple syrup (optional)

**Directions:**

Bring water and milk to a boil, slowly whisk in buckwheat, salt and spices. Turn heat on low to simmer, stirring often over the next 10 minutes. Remove from burner and stir in pumpkin and nut butter until well blended. Can be served as a complete meal or separated into smaller portions for when that is better tolerated. Double the recipe and refrigerate for up to three days for a delicious quick meal or snack.

# Veggie Sides

## Moroccan Spiced Sweet Potatoes
**Ingredients:**

- 1 sweet potato, peeled and diced into ½- to 1-inch cubes
- Olive or coconut oil, or butter if the oils are too heavy to start out with (you'll want to try them later when you are able to eat more)
- Moroccan Spice Blend (see recipe below for these spices that support digestion, not just make food taste delicious)

**Directions:**

Mix spices in a small bowl. One teaspoon at a time, sprinkle potatoes with spices, about half the mix. For stronger flavors, feel free to generously coat them. Place in a steamer basket over boiling water in saucepan, then cover and simmer 10 to 15 minutes, or until fork tender. Remove, and, if tolerated, drizzle with a teaspoon of olive or coconut oil before serving.

**If you do not have a steamer basket:** Combine diced and spiced sweet potato with 2 to 3 teaspoons oil, place in baking dish, cover with foil, and bake for 15 to 20 minutes at 400 degrees.

Feel free to substitute other vegetables such as winter squash, carrots, parsnips, white potatoes or a combination of your favorites.

## Moroccan Spice Blend

**Ingredients:**

- 1 teaspoon ground coriander
- 1 teaspoon ground cumin
- 1 teaspoon paprika
- ½ teaspoon cinnamon
- ¼ teaspoon Himalayan salt
- ⅛ teaspoon ground ginger (optional)

This spice blend includes some wonderful digestive aids and releases a sweet, exotic aroma in the air.

*Tip! If you enjoy this spice combo, triple the ingredients and store in a small jar for future use. This blend complements many dishes including rice, chicken, fish and hot cereals for breakfast.*

## Zucchini Ribbons and Summer Sauce

Makes 4 to 6 servings

**Ingredients:**

- 4 to 5 medium zucchini
- 1 tablespoon olive oil
- 1 teaspoon dried oregano or Herbs de Provence (depending on taste preference)
- ½ teaspoon sea salt
- ¼-½ cup vegetable or chicken broth (optional for sauce). Remember, the cleaner, the better.

**Directions:**

Preheat oven to 375 degrees. Wash zucchini and begin by chopping off the rough end. Peel dark, outside layer first and discard. Next, peel long, thin ribbons and stop when seeds begin to appear. Continue to work around until all that is left is the seeded, middle part. Once each one is finished, place ribbons in a small baking dish. Drizzle with olive oil and mix in seasonings. Finally, cover with foil and allow to cook for 30 minutes, softly stirring halfway through. The zucchini will release its own juices and create steam that seals in the flavors.

This is excellent as a side dish, but can also be made into a smooth, creamy sauce. Just add broth, a little at a time, in blender, until desired consistency is achieved. This is a wonderful addition to pasta, rice, baked potato, on fish or chicken, or even on its own. Freeze any leftover sauce in ice cube trays to save and add to soups.

# Pancakes Two Ways

## Sprouted Pancakes for Everyone

Spelt has many benefits, and those sensitive to wheat can often tolerate this ancient grain. You may be surprised by how well it's digested and how delicious it tastes; similar to regular flour with a slight nutty flavor.

The benefits of sprouted flour:

- Easier to digest: Sprouting breaks down the starches in grains into simple sugars so your body can digest them like a vegetable (like a tomato, not a potato).

- Increased vitamin C: Sprouting produces vitamin C.

- Increased vitamin B: Sprouting increases the vitamin B content (B2, B5 and B6).

- Increased carotene: Sprouting increases the carotene up to eight times.

- Increased enzymes are produced during sprouting.

- Reduction of anti-nutrients: Sprouting neutralizes enzyme inhibitors and phytic acid, which is a substance present in the bran of all grains that inhibits absorption of calcium, magnesium, iron, copper and zinc.

We suggest Shiloh Farms brand, as we are impressed with their long history and their promise of foods that are "pure and wholesome, no artificial ingredients, no preservatives and only natural flavor."

If you are worried about spending the extra money on this special flour, we understand where you are coming from. However, if you suffer from any digestive problems, nothing is more important than giving yourself the most nutrient-dense, easy-to-digest fuel available. In fact, if you break it down, a 5-pound bag, for example, would make you and your family pancakes once a week for more than four months. That equates to approximately $2 a week, (about $5 with other ingredients), for a nutrient-dense and delicious meal. It really helps to appreciate the cost versus benefit.

*Notes:*

- *Individuals with wheat-related conditions like celiac sprue or gluten-sensitive enteropathies, should consult with their healthcare practitioner before experimenting with any of the "gluten grains," including spelt.*

- *If you are sensitive to corn, you can eliminate it completely and replace it with spelt flour.*

- *Though we highly recommend using the sprouted spelt flour, it can be replaced with regular flour or a gluten-free flour mix, if you prefer.*

**Ingredients:**

- 1 cup Shiloh Farms Sprouted Spelt Flour
- ½ cup organic sprouted corn flour, can be blue
- ¼ cup pure coconut sugar, or organic sugar
- 1¼ teaspoon baking powder
- ¼ teaspoon baking soda
- ¼ teaspoon salt
- 1 cup plain kefir or yogurt diluted with ¼ cup water. (Suggestions for yogurt are: Latta USA yogurt, White Mountain Bulgarian Yogurt or Stonyfield)

- 4 tablespoons coconut oil and/or butter
- 2 egg yolks + 2 egg whites, separated, cage-free, humanely raised, no chemicals
- 1 teaspoon finely grated lemon zest
- ½-1 cup blueberries, frozen or fresh
- Pure maple syrup

**Directions:**

Mix dry and wet ingredients (minus egg whites), in two separate bowls with whisk. Pour wet over dry and gently whisk until just combined. Beat egg whites until there are peaks, stiff, but not dry, and fold into batter. Heat large skillet over medium heat and allow to warm. Lightly spray with oil or spread enough to just moisten pan. Drop in ¼-cup scoops of batter, adding blueberries to some, and allow to cook long enough to lightly brown bottom, until edges just begin to form (about 2 to 3 minutes). Flip and cook another 1 or 2 minutes, until golden. Place in oven at 200 degrees to keep warm while finishing batch.

Serve and top with blueberries and pure maple syrup.

While following our New Approach, in time you may be able to tolerate more foods such as blueberries, raspberries and strawberries.

*Tip! If you are low in energy and looking for a pancake mix and do not have an intolerance to gluten, then a good mix suggestion is Arrowhead Mills Organic Sprouted Grain Pancake & Waffle Mix. Arrowhead Mills also offers a gluten-free option for pre-mix pancakes that many have been able to tolerate well. It is suggested to use coconut milk instead of regular milk or water.*

## Pumpkin Pancakes

Pumpkin is an excellent source of vitamin A (1 cup has 760 percent of the daily recommended value!) as well as vitamin C, iron and calcium. The ways to use pumpkin are endless, for example adding a scoop to hot cereal, smoothies, soup, etc. This recipe for a protein-rich breakfast creates a light and fluffy crepe-like pancake, with plenty of fall flavor.

Adapted from Practical Paleo
Makes 2 GP servings

### Ingredients:

- 2 eggs (1 egg + 2 whites if wanting to lower the fat content)
- ¼ cup canned pumpkin, organic
- ½ teaspoon pure vanilla extract, organic
- 1 tablespoon maple syrup (optional)
- ½ teaspoon pumpkin pie spice
- ½ teaspoon cinnamon
- ⅛ teaspoon salt
- ⅛ teaspoon baking soda
- Coconut oil

### Directions:

Whisk eggs, pumpkin, vanilla and maple syrup together. Sift spices and baking soda into the wet ingredients. Melt a small amount of coconut oil over medium heat and allow it to lightly spread over the pan. Spoon batter in skillet to make pancakes of desired size. When bubbles appear, flip once to finish cooking. Serve with yogurt for a nice breakfast or as a snack.

# SHARED EXPERIENCES

## Stephanie's Journey with Gastroparesis

*I was diagnosed with gastroparesis (GP) at the age of 28, following months of feeling like I had the flu. The "radiated egg" (gastric emptying study) confirmed the slow motility of my stomach.*

*I had lived with digestive issues on and off from the age of 19, shortly after undergoing laparoscopic surgery for endometriosis and ovarian cysts. It started with heartburn and eventually symptoms that were diagnosed as IBS. At the time, I thought I could cure it through diet alone and went completely gluten free. For about six months I felt amazing but it didn't last and I began experiencing severe bloating, fullness, nausea and eventually it became difficult to even keep down fluids. Two months later I was in the hospital having every test in the book done.*

*With motility medication, bodywork, rest and loads of support from family and friends, I began to recover and was ready to get my life back. One year later I enrolled at Bastyr University and began a full-time course in acupuncture and Chinese medicine. The program was incredible, a dream come true, but traveling the 90 miles back and forth each week, missing my husband, not to mention the time and stress involved with the intense studies, became more than I could handle. By the end of the first year I had lost a tremendous amount of weight, in denial of having a chronic illness because I was determined to live a "normal" life.*

*By June 2010, I ended up back in the hospital, this time too weak and malnourished to recover on my own. After unsuccessful trials with medications as well as a round of Botox treatments, I had no choice but to be put on a temporary feeding tube, also known as a j-tube. This is when it really hit me...it was time to accept my illness and really focus on taking care of myself because otherwise I wouldn't survive much longer.*

By accepting this condition as part of my life, I was able to slow down and set priorities. I again started focusing on managing symptoms through diet, exercise, limiting stress and finding other passions in life like creativity and helping others. I still had bad days, but I learned how to manage them by not letting the fear take over and by not running away from them.

I began blogging about my journey, learning more and more about GP and how many others were going through similar battles. Motivated to help, I enrolled in a program through the Institute for Integrative Nutrition to become certified as a health coach. In June 2012, I started to use my experience and education as a learning tool for others, to focus on the things we can do to help ourselves instead of focusing on the things we can't.

I never would have imagined this would be my life at this age but it hasn't stopped me from continuing to stay positive, be an advocate for awareness and, in the meantime, live the best life possible.

Little did I know how much crazier life would get!

Due to complications, in the fall of 2012 the j-tube was removed. Unfortunately, my body did not hold onto the calories I was able to take in and after a drastic weight loss, another tube was placed in January 2013. The complications only increased, resulting in having a PICC line for IV nutrition placed in February 2013. After insisting for six months that the second j-tube was causing more harm than good because I was unable to tolerate any feeds, it was removed through a laparoscopic procedure.

The PICC line was eventually replaced with a central line in my chest for a more permanent solution and by 2015 with a port-a-cath due to the lines not staying in properly. I'm still able to eat and try to focus on nutrient-dense foods but it still is not the amount my body requires. For now, TPN (total parenteral nutrition) continues to be used five nights a week.

*For the last few years, I have been lucky enough to work as a nutrition consumer advocate for ThriveRx and support those in similar situations all around the country. In addition, along with a fantastic volunteer team, we have organized the Awareness Walk for Gastroparesis and Digestive Health for four years now, raising not only awareness for our disorder, but funds to go toward research specifically for gastroparesis.*

*Just recently I was introduced to Chalyce and Essential7 and began researching all that she has done for herself and for others. By using her custom essential oil GP Starter Collection, in just a few short weeks I went from eating two small meals a day to three, with fewer challenges than before. Of course, this doesn't mean that suddenly I'm all better, but it gives me hope that one day I could feel an even bigger difference. The essential oils are more powerful than I ever expected and after reading testimonials from others whose lives have greatly improved, I am excited to continue this journey, share it with others and see where it all goes.*

# APPENDIX

## The Chemistry of Essential Oils

Chalyce had the pleasure of listening to Dr. David Stewart speak in her early years of learning about essential oils through Young Living conventions. Not only does Dr. Stewart cite science-based research, he also traces essential oils to the Bible. Did you know that essential oils are mentioned 1,031 times in the Bible? That is pretty powerful as you can imagine it as the first reference guide to essential oils.

Here we share Dr. Stewart's quick course in chemistry to give you a better understanding of why essential oils are so powerful.

### A Quick Course in Chemistry
*By Dr. David Stewart*

Because of the tiny molecular structure of the components of an essential oil, they are extremely concentrated. One drop contains approximately 40 million-trillion molecules. Numerically that is a 4 with 19 zeros after it: 40,000,000,000,000,000,000. We have 100 trillion cells in our bodies, and that's a lot. But one drop of essential oil contains enough molecules to cover every cell in our bodies with 40,000 molecules. Considering that it only takes one molecule of the right kind to open a receptor site and communicate with the DNA to alter cellular function, you can see why even inhaling a small amount of oil vapor can have profound effects on the body, brain and emotions. Sometimes too many oil molecules overload the receptor sites, and they freeze up without responding at all when a smaller amount would have been just right. This is why we say that when using oils, "sometimes less is better."

Sometimes more is better, too. Knowing the difference is the art of aromatherapy.

Essential oils are mixtures of dozens, even hundreds, of constituents, all of which are composed of carbon and hydrogen and sometimes oxygen. All essential oils are principally composed of a class of organic compounds built of "isoprene units."

An isoprene unit is a set of five connected carbon atoms with eight hydrogens attached. Their molecular weight is only 68 amu, which is very small, indeed. Molecules built of isoprene units are all classified as "terpenes." Terpenes are what make essential oils unique in the world of natural substances.

## Phenylpropanoids

Phenylpropanoids are compounds of carbon-ring molecules, incorporating one isoprene unit. They are also called hemiterpenes. There are dozens of varieties of phenylpropanoids. They are found in clove (90 percent), cassia (80 percent), basil (75 percent), cinnamon (73 percent), oregano (60 percent), anise (50 percent), peppermint (25 percent). While they can create conditions where unfriendly viruses and bacteria cannot live, the most important function performed by phenylpropanoids is that they clean the receptor sites on the cells. Without clean receptor sites, cells cannot communicate, and the body malfunctions, resulting in sickness.

## Monoterpenes

Monoterpenes are compounds of two isoprene units, which is 10 carbon atoms and 16 hydrogen atoms per molecule-molecular weight 136 amu. There are an estimated 2,000 varieties of monoterpenes.

Monoterpenes are found in most essential oils: galbanum (80 percent), angelica (73 percent), hyssop (70 percent), rose of

Sharon (54 percent), peppermint (45 percent), juniper (42 percent), frankincense (40 percent), spruce (38 percent), pine (30 percent), cypress (28 percent) and myrtle (25 percent).

While offering a variety of healing properties, the most important ability of the monoterpenes is that they can reprogram miswritten information in the cellular memory. With improper coding in the DNA, cells malfunction and diseases result, including lethal ones such as cancer.

## Sesquiterpenes

Sesquiterpenes are compounds of three isoprene units, which is 15 carbons and 24 hydrogens per molecule, with a molecular weight of 204 amu. There are more than 10,000 kinds of sesquiterpenes. Sesquiterpenes are the principal constituents of cedarwood (98 percent), vetiver (97 percent), spikenard (93 percent), sandalwood (aloes) (90 percent), black pepper (74 percent), patchouli (71 percent), myrrh (62 percent) and ginger (59 percent). They are also found in galbanum, onycha and frankincense (8 percent).

Sesquiterpene molecules deliver oxygen molecules to cells, like hemoglobin does in the blood. Sesquiterpenes can also erase or deprogram miswritten codes in the DNA. Sesquiterpenes are thought to be especially effective in fighting cancer because the root problem with a cancer cell is that it contains misinformation, and sesquiterpenes can erase that garbled information. At the same time, the oxygen carried by sesquiterpene molecules creates an environment where cancer cells can't reproduce.

Hence, sesquiterpenes deliver cancer cells a double punch—one that disables their coded misbehavior and a second that stops their growth. The American Medical Association (AMA) has said that if they could find an agent that would pass the blood-brain barrier, they would be able to find cures for ailments such as Lou Gehrig's disease, multiple sclerosis, Alzheimer's disease and Parkinson's disease. Such agents already exist and have been available since Biblical times. The agents, of course, are essential oils, particularly those containing the brain-oxygenating molecules of sesquiterpenes.

## The Triple Whammy

The big triple punch combination of "PMS" (phenylpropanoids, monoterpenes and sesquiterpenes) found in essential oils is very powerful in addressing many illnesses, injuries and disease conditions. That is because this combination offers the following:

- First, the receptor sites are cleaned, allowing the proper transfer of hormones, peptides, neurotransmitters, steroids and other intracellular messengers. (The phenylpropanoids do that.)

- Second, cellular memory stored in the DNA is de-programmed and wrong information is erased. (The sesquiterpenes take care of that.)

- Third, you reprogram the cells with the correct information so they can function properly. (The monoterpenes do this.)

These three classes of chemical components are why essential oils can sometimes affect a healing process that is nearly instant and also permanent. What they simply do is to restore the body back to its natural state of balance and health. While a specific oil may have one or two of these three classes of compounds as its predominant chemistry, all the Biblical oils contain some or all of them. This is one secret to their amazing healing abilities.

So there you have it, in a nutshell, the way the blood-brain barrier works and the biochemistry of one of the ways essential oils can help achieve healing.

More information about Dr. David Stewart can be found at www.carepublications.net/authors/david_stewart.html

# All About Coconut Oil

Dr. Bruce Fife is a leading expert in the use of coconut for health and healing. The following information is from his research site and used with written permission:

Coconut water has been a popular beverage in the tropics for generations, and it wasn't long before physicians began experimenting with it for oral rehydration. They found that it was just as effective orally as it was intravenously in combating dehydration. Due to coconut water's chemical composition, it is absorbed through the intestinal wall quicker than plain water, bringing about a faster recovery and eliminating the need for IV rehydration therapy.

Today, coconut water is used worldwide as a home treatment for dehydration-related diseases such as cholera and influenza. Cholera, which is a major health problem in many underdeveloped countries, is characterized by severe diarrhea and vomiting. Death rates from cholera are high. Death, however, is not caused by the infection itself, but by dehydration, resulting from the loss of body fluids. Giving cholera patients adequate amounts of coconut water results in a remarkable 97 percent recovery rate.

One of the secrets to coconut water's success as a rehydration fluid is its mineral or electrolyte content. Coconut water contains the same major electrolytes as those in human body fluids. When we lose water from diarrhea or perspiration, we also lose electrolytes. It is necessary to replace both water and electrolytes. Coconut water does this, plain water does not. For this reason, coconut water has recently become popular as a natural sports hydration beverage. Some people call it "Nature's Gatorade," but it is far better than Gatorade.

In hot weather, or during heavy physical activity, we lose a substantial amount of water as sweat. Not only do you lose water, but you also lose electrolytes, particularly sodium and potassium. Electrolytes are essential for energy production and nerve and muscle function. Our bodies require precise amounts of each electrolyte. The loss of just 6 percent of potassium, for instance, can cause heart failure. So maintaining proper electrolyte levels is essential. When we become dehydrated, we are generally deficient in electrolytes as well. Drinking water may replenish the lost fluids, but not the electrolytes. An athlete who loses a lot of water and does not adequately replenish electrolytes will experience muscle cramping, weakness, nausea, vomiting, diarrhea, and eventually go into a coma and may die. Electrolyte deficiency is one of the biggest dangers athletes face, particularly for those who participate in endurance races such as marathons and triathlons.

It may seem obvious to drink when the weather is hot or during heavy physical activity, but many people underestimate the magnitude of their fluid loss. It is very difficult to avoid dehydration during a long race, or when working in the heat, because the rate of sweat loss usually exceeds the rate of absorption of ingested fluids. The maximum rate of fluid absorption by the gastrointestinal tract during exercise is approximately 27 ounces per hour. The rate of fluid loss through sweating can easily reach 1 liter (34 ounces) per hour and can soar to 2 liters per hour under very strenuous conditions. If you lose 34 ounces of sweat and drink an equal amount of water, you will still become dehydrated because the body can only absorb 27 ounces. Thus, it is not possible to drink enough to stay hydrated, and dehydration will still occur despite drinking plenty of fluid.

Drinking only water, without a source of electrolytes, can dilute the electrolytes in your bloodstream, causing a serious electrolyte deficiency. Many athletes have been sent to the hospital for this very reason.

The problem with commercial sports drinks, however, is that their electrolyte content is too low to be of much benefit. Sodium and chloride (salt) are usually the only electrolytes they contain.

Potassium, another essential electrolyte that is lost, is often not even included. Commercial sports drinks also contain various questionable additives such as chemical dyes, emulsifiers and preservatives. Basically, these popular sports drinks are nothing more than non-carbonated soft drinks with a little added salt. Contrary to popular opinion and marketing hype, these drinks are not recommended for preventing serious dehydration.

Coconut water offers a superior option to commercial sports drinks. Unlike these other beverages, coconut water is recommended for rehydration. Coconut water is completely natural with no harmful chemical additives. Unlike sports drinks, it contains all the major electrolytes important to the human body—sodium, potassium, chloride, magnesium, calcium, phosphate and sulfate, as well as important trace minerals such as zinc and selenium, and contains more potassium than a banana. It also supplies other important nutrients missing from sports drinks, such as amino acids, vitamins and antioxidants, all of which support a healthy body and proper hydration.

Coconut water has proven to be a superior rehydration fluid when taken both intravenously and orally. It is completely compatible with the human body as demonstrated by being injected directly into the bloodstream without any harmful effect. Can you imagine the damage that would occur if you tried to inject Gatorade into your bloodstream? The purpose of consuming rehydration beverages is to replace fluids and nutrients lost from the blood, so it is only logical to use a product that can do this effectively and harmlessly.

My book, *Coconut Water for Health and Healing*, describes the many health benefits of this remarkable beverage. It includes a fascinating account of how coconut water has been used as an emergency IV fluid around the world and why it is becoming one of the most popular sports rehydration drinks today.

Coconut water isn't just for rehydration, however. Studies show it provides numerous health benefits, some of which are the following: dissolving kidney stones, protecting against cancer, balancing blood sugar, providing ionic trace minerals, improving digestion, feeding friendly gut bacteria, relieving constipation, reducing risk of heart disease, improving blood circulation, lowering high blood pressure, helping prevent atherosclerosis, possessing anti-aging properties, and enhancing immune function.

Coconut water tastes delicious straight from the coconut, but can also serve as the base for a variety of foods and beverages. Included are 36 tantalizing coconut water recipes. With 80 percent less sugar than fruit juice or soda, coconut water makes a healthy, refreshing drink for you and your kids.

## Coconut (Cocos Nucifera): The Tree of Life

The scientific name for coconut is Cocos nucifera. Early Spanish explorers called it coco, which means "monkey face" because the three indentations (eyes) on the hairy nut resembles the head and face of a monkey. Nucifera means "nut-bearing."

The coconut provides a nutritious source of meat, juice, milk and oil that has fed and nourished populations around the world for generations. On many islands, coconut is a staple in the diet and provides the majority of the food eaten. Nearly one-third of the world's population depends on the coconut, to some degree, for their food and their economy. Among these cultures, the coconut has a long and respected history. Coconut is highly nutritious and rich in fiber, vitamins and minerals. It is classified as a "functional food" because it provides many health benefits beyond its nutritional content. Coconut oil is of special interest because it possesses healing properties far beyond that of any other dietary oil and is extensively used in traditional medicine among Asian and Pacific populations. Pacific Islanders consider coconut oil to be the cure for all illness. The coconut palm is so highly valued by them as both a source of food and medicine that it is called "The Tree of Life." Only recently has modern medical science unlocked the secrets to coconut's amazing healing powers.

## Coconut in Traditional Medicine

People from many diverse cultures, languages, religions and races, scattered around the globe, have revered the coconut as a valuable source of both food and medicine. Wherever the coconut palm grows, the people have learned of its importance as an effective medicine.

For thousands of years, coconut products have held a respected and valuable place in local folk medicine.

In traditional medicine around the world, coconut is used to treat a wide variety of health problems including the following: abscesses, asthma, baldness, bronchitis, bruises, burns, colds, constipation, cough, dropsy, dysentery, earache, fever, flu, gingivitis, gonorrhea, irregular or painful menstruation, jaundice, kidney stones, lice, malnutrition, nausea, rash, scabies, scurvy, skin infections, sore throat, swelling, syphilis, toothache, tuberculosis, tumors, typhoid, ulcers, upset stomach, weakness and wounds.

## Coconut in Modern Medicine

Modern medical science is now confirming the use of coconut in treating many of the above conditions. Published studies in medical journals show that coconut, in one form or another, may provide a wide range of health benefits. Some of these are summarized below:

- Improves digestion and absorption of other nutrients including vitamins, minerals and amino acids.
- Provides a nutritional source of quick energy.
- Relieves stress on pancreas and enzyme systems of the body.
- Reduces symptoms associated with pancreatitis.
- Helps to relieve symptoms and reduce health risks associated with diabetes.
- Reduces problems associated with malabsorption syndrome and cystic fibrosis.
- Improves calcium and magnesium absorption and supports the development of strong bones and teeth.
- Helps protect against osteoporosis.
- Helps to relieve symptoms associated with gallbladder disease.
- Relieves symptoms associated with Crohn's disease, ulcerative colitis and stomach ulcers.
- Improves digestion and bowel function.
- Relieves pain and irritation caused by hemorrhoids.
- Reduces inflammation.
- Supports tissue healing and repair.

*This material was used with permission from the author, Dr. Bruce Fife, ND (www.coconutresearchcenter.org). For more information about Dr. Fife's book Coconut Water for Health and Healing, visit www.piccadillybooks.com.*

# Suggested Products

**Coconut Water**

Big Tree Farms, 541-488-5605, www.bigtreefarms.com

CocoHydro powder, www.bigtreefarms.com/products/coco-hydro

Harvest Bay, www.harvest-bay.com/content/harvest-bay-home

Amy and Brian, www.amyandbriannaturals.com

Harmless Harvest, www.harmlessharvest.com

**Essential Oils**

Essential7, www.essential7.com

**Kefir Grains**

Kefir Lady, 517-610-8366, www.kefirlady.com

**Kefir/Yogurt**

Latta USA, www.lattausa.com (May be available in supermarkets such as Whole Foods Northern California, Wegmans, Sprouts, Shop Rite, A&P)

Stonyfield Greek Organic Whole Milk Yogurt, 800-776-2697, www.stonyfield.com/products/yogurt/whole-milk-greek/plain

B'More Organic Skyr Smoothie, 410-417-7579, www.bmoreorganic.com

## Moringa

Organic India, 888-550-8332, www.organicindiausa.com/organic-india-moringa-capsules/

## Protein Bars

Amazing Grass Bars, 866-472-7711, www.amazinggrass.com
GoMacro Bars, 800-788-9540, www.gomacro.com

## Protein Powder/Shakes/Beverages

Garden of Life Organic Plant Protein, 866-465-0051, www.gardenoflife.com/products-for-life-category/product-families/organic-plant-protein

Orgain, www.orgain.com

Plant Fusion Protein, 800-848-0089, www.plantfusion.net

R.W. Knudsen Recharge Drink, www.rwknudsenfamily.com/products/recharge

Stomach Ease Tea - Yogi Teas, 800-964-4832, www.yogiproducts.com/teas/stomach-ease/

SunWarrior Organic Protein Warrior Blend, 888-540-3667, www.sunwarrior.com

## Sprouted Spelt Flour

Shiloh Farms, 800-362-6832 x103, www.shilohfarms.com

# Online Resources

Essential7 Oils, www.essential7.com

Healing Gastroparesis Naturally, www.healinggpnaturaly.info

Healing Gastroparesis Naturally Facebook Group, www.facebook.com/groups/667046093329732/

Journey with Gastroparesis Blog, www.mygastroparesisjourney.blogspot.com

Patreon, www.patreon.com/healinggp

# References

## Chapter 1

"Gastroparesis." National Institutes of Health. U.S. Department of Health and Human Services, June 2012. Web.

Digestive Health Team. "Gastroparesis: Know the Risk Factors for This Mysterious Stomach Condition." Health Essentials from Cleveland Clinic. N.p., 08 Sept. 2015. Web.

"Healing." Wikipedia. Wikimedia Foundation. https://en.wikipedia.org/wiki/Healing

Mullin, Gerard E., and Kathie Madonna. Swift. *The Inside Tract: Your Good Gut Guide to Great Digestive Health*. New York, NY: Rodale, 2011. 101-102

"Gastroparesis - NORD (National Organization for Rare Disorders)." NORD National Organization for Rare Disorders Gastroparesis. 2009, 2012. http://rarediseases.org/rare-diseases/gastroparesis/

U.S. Food and Drug Administration. "FDA Approves Breath Test to Aid in Diagnosis of Delayed Gastric Emptying." 7 Apr. 2015. http://www.fda.gov/NewsEvents/Newsroom/PressAnnouncements/ucm441370.htm

## Chapter 2

Devries, Stephen R. "Doctors Need to Learn About Nutrition." Medscape. 4 Sept. 2014. http://www.medscape.com/viewarticle/830697.

Aridogan, BC. "Antimicrobial Activity and Chemical Composition of Some Essential Oils." Archives of Pharmacal Research. U.S. National Library of Medicine, 25 Dec. 2002. Web.

Aggarwal, Bharat B., and Debora Yost. *Healing Spices: How to Use 50 Everyday and Exotic Spices to Boost Health and Beat Disease*. New York: Sterling Pub., 2011.

Taylor, Leslie. *The Healing Power of Rainforest Herbs: A Guide to Understanding and Using Herbal Medicinals*. Garden City Park, NY: Square One, 2005.

Stewart, David. *The Chemistry of Essential Oils Made Simple*. Marble Hill: Care Publications, 2005.

Ehrlich, Steven D. "Peppermint." University of Maryland Medical Center. N.p., 6 July 2014. http://umm.edu/health/medical/altmed/herb/peppermint

"Essential Oils." Organic Facts. https://www.organicfacts.net/health-benefits/essential-oils

**Chapter 3**

REINAGEL, MONICA, MS, LD/N, CNS. "Kefir: From Russia with Love." Food & Nutrition. N.p., 3 June 2014. Web

Parrish, Carol Rees, and Jeanne Keith-Ferris. "Diet Intervention for Gastroparesis." UVA Nutrition Services. https://uvahealth.com/services/digestive-health/images-and-docs/gastroparesis-diet.pdf

Suttie, Emma. "The Spleen." Chinese Medicine Living. N.p., 27 June 2012. https://www.chinesemedicineliving.com/medicine/organs/the-spleen/

Plotner, Becky. "Sauerkraut Test Divulges Shocking Probiotic Count." Nourishing Plot. 21 June 2014.

"Can Too Much Sauerkraut Damage Your Thyroid?" Nourished and Nurtured. 22 May 2011. http://nourishedandnurtured.blogspot.com/2011/05/thyroid-goitrogens-and-recipe-for.html

Daniel, Kaayla. "Why Broth Is Beautiful: Essential Roles for Proline, Glycine and Gelatin - Weston A Price." Weston A Price. N.p., 18 June 2003. http://www.westonaprice.org/health-topics/why-broth-is-beautiful-essential-roles-for-proline-glycine-and-gelatin/

"Probiotics and Their Fermented Food Products are Beneficial for Health." National Center for Biotechnology Information. U.S. National Library of Medicine, June 2006. http://www.ncbi.nlm.nih.gov/ pubmed/16696665

Fallon, Sally, and Mary G. Enig. *Nourishing Traditions: The Cookbook That Challenges Politically Correct Nutrition and the Diet Dictocrats.* Brandywine, MD: NewTrends Pub., 2001. 100

"Debunking The Salt Myth: Add This Seasoning to Food Daily." Mercola.com. 20 Sept. 2011. http://articles.mercola.com/sites/articles/archive/2011/09/20/salt-myth.aspx

**Chapter** 4

Mullin, Gerard E. "Yoga and Digestive Health." Integrative Gastroenterology. New York: Oxford UP, 2011. 350-51.

Nakazawa, Donna Jackson. *The Last Best Cure: My Quest to Awaken the Healing Parts of My Brain-and Get Back My Body, My Joy, and My Life.* New York, NY: Hudson Street, 2013. 186-87.

Pavlov, Valentin A., Hong Wang, Christopher J. Czura, Steven G. Friedman, and Kevin J. Tracey. "The Cholinergic Anti-inflammatory Pathway: A Missing Link in Neuroimmunomodulation." Molecular Medicine. ScholarOne, Aug. 2003. http://www.ncbi.nlm.nih.gov/pmc/articles/PMC1430829/

SAGE Publications. "Could Rosemary Scent Boost Brain Performance?" ScienceDaily. 24 February 2012. www.sciencedaily.com/releases/2012/02/120224194313.htm

Sloan, RP, H. McCreath, KJ Tracey, S. Sidney, K. Liu, and T. Seeman. "RR Interval Variability Is Inversely Related to Inflammatory Markers: The CARDIA Study." National Center for Biotechnology Information. U.S. National Library of Medicine, Apr. 2007. http://www.ncbi.nlm.nih.gov/pubmed/17592552

Wenk, Gary Lee. *Your Brain on Food: How Chemicals Control Your Thoughts and Feelings.* Oxford UP, 2010.

Petersen, Angela Savitri. "Activating the Vagus Nerve." Eiri Eolas Blog. 15 June 2013. http://eiriu-eolas.org/2013/06/15/activating-the-vagus-nerve/

Mayo Clinic Staff. "Stress Management." Relaxation Techniques: Try These Steps to Reduce Stress. http://www.mayoclinic.org/relaxation-technique/art-20045368

Rakel, David. UW Integrative Medicine Program Dept. of Family Medicine, University of Wisconsin-Madison. "Improving and Maintaining a Healthy Sleep-Wake Cycle" Patient Handout. March 2008

Rattana, Guru. "Sa Ta Na Ma Meditation for Evolutionary Change." Kundalini Yoga. http://www.kundaliniyoga.org/kyt15.html

## Chapter 5

Abaci, M.D. Peter. "A Radical Shift to Better Pain Relief." The Huffington Post. TheHuffingtonPost.com, 05 Dec. 2012. Web.

"Moringa: Uses, Side Effects, Interactions and Warnings." WebMD http://www.webmd.com/vitamins-supplements/ingredientmo-no-1242-moringa.aspx?activeingredientid=1242

Bernier, Julie. "The Art of Drinking Water: 10 Ayurvedic Tips for a Happy Hydrated Body." Elephant Journal. 30 Oct. 2013. http://www. elephantjournal.com/2013/10/the-art-of-drinking-water-10-ayurvedic-tips-for-a-happily-hydrated-body-julie-bernier/

## Chapter 6

Beim, Mim. "Five Emotions That Make You Sick." My Body+Soul. http://www.bodyandsoul.com.au/health/health+advice/five+emotions+that+make+you+sick,12099

Rankin, Lissa. "Redefining Health." *Mind over Medicine: Scientific Proof That You Can Heal Yourself.* Hay House, 2013. 71.

"The Definition of Affirmation." Dictionary.com. http://www.dictionary.com/browse/affirmation

"The Emotions." Chinese Medicine Living. N.p., 17 July 2012. https://www.chinesemedicineliving.com/philosophy/the-emotions/

Chandler, Cynthia K. *Animal Assisted Therapy in Counseling.* New York: Routledge, 2005.

Lipton, Bruce H. *The Biology of Belief: Unleashing the Power of Consciousness, Matter and Miracles.* Santa Rosa, CA: Mountain of Love/Elite, 2005.

Dyer, Wayne W. *Excuses Begone! How to Change Lifelong, Self-Defeating Thinking Habits.* Carlsbad, CA: Hay House, 2009.

## Chapter 7

Wallace, Carey. "3 Reasons Your Daughter's Puberty Won't Be Like Yours." Time. 9 Jan. 2015. http://time.com/3659760/3-reasons-your-daughters-puberty-wont-be-like-yours/

Worwood, Valerie Ann. *Aromatherapy for the Healthy Child: More Than 300 Natural, Nontoxic, and Fragrant Essential Oil Blends.* Novato, CA: New World Library, 2000.

"Top 5 Websites for Healthy and Organic Recipes for Kids." Green and Clean Mom. 23 June 2011. http://greenandcleanmom.org/top-5-websites-for-healthy-and-organic-recipes-for-kids/

## Chapter 8

Gokani, MD Trupti. "The Gut-Brain Link: How Your Headaches Might Stem From Your Digestion." TheHuffingtonPost.com, 13 Jan. 2015. http://www.huffingtonpost.com/trupti-gokani-md/the-gut-brain-link-how-you_b_6097774.html

Swanson, Jerry W. "Migraines and Gastrointestinal Problems: Is There a Link?" Mayo Clinic. 16 Oct. 2015. http://www.mayoclinic.org/diseases-conditions/migraine-headache/expert-answers/migraines/faq-20058268

"Headache Triggers." Cigna. http://www.cignabehavioral.com/web/basicsite/bulletinBoard/headacheTriggers.jsp

## Chapter 9

Bieler, Henry G. *Food Is Your Best Medicine*. New York: Random House, 1966.

Fallon, Sally, and Mary G. Enig. *Nourishing Traditions: The Cookbook That Challenges Politically Correct Nutrition and the Diet Dictocrats*. Brandywine, MD: NewTrends Pub., 2001. 112-113

## Appendix

Fife, Bruce. "Coconut Research Center." Coconut Research Center. http://coconutresearchcenter.org/

# Acknowledgments

**Chalyce's acknowledgements:**

I would like to thank all the volunteers and donors who helped make this book happen; without you, our book would never have been published. To Joanne Ramsey for making the first donation towards the book.

Kathleen and Lynette, for having faith and trust in me, without you both, our GP family would never have been created.

To my parents, James and Pat, Nancy and Dennis, my brother Reese, all of my cousins and friends who have supported me and let me throw my "chicken bones" and do my "voodoo" since I was a teenager. Thank you for believing in me and encouraging me to stay on my path even though it was very crooked at times.

To my children, Staige and Jasna, for understanding when I travel to help others, for their tender hearts and love that they show others. For the hours sitting and helping with my clients, making their day a little brighter with your smiles.

Many, many thanks to "Doc" (Dr. Patricia Williams), for saving my life and my son Staige's, and for starting me on this path 30 years ago. I wish you were here to see how far I have come with the knowledge you shared with me. Your wisdom and kindness stays in my heart forever.

My spiritual teachers, Dr. Lynn Crocker and Sevak Singh Khalsa, who guide and support me on my path of healing my traumatic brain disorder (TBI). Without Kundalini Yoga, I would still be challenged. Sat Nam and Wahe Guru—thank you for keeping me keeping up. To Stephanie who is key to making this all flow together, putting meaning behind my research, putting into words my very thoughts.

I dedicate this book to my family members who have crossed the path to the other side. My sweet sister Chauntelle who has been my driving force from the heavens above. My stepfather Dennis who encourages me every day to shine bright. My Aunt Nancy and Uncle James who have blessed me every day with their generosity and support that will last for years to come. Thank you for being a part of my life, I am so blessed to have all of you.

**Stephanie's acknowledgments:**

I would like to thank everyone who has supported me over the years, whether that be as simple as a phone call or a hug, making nourishing soups when I was too sick to do so on my own, and being that shoulder to cry on.

A big thank you to Trevor, who has stood by me through more than I ever thought possible and never once thought there was any other way. Who does so well at reminding me of the importance of self-care when I'm up writing for hours or scheming ways to travel the world!

To my closest friends and family, I am incredibly blessed to be surrounded by such caring and incredible beings.

To all of the medical professionals, both traditional and non-traditional, who haven't given up on me.

To this amazing woman who came into my life at just the right time: Chalyce, thank you for so generously sharing your experience and guidance, and allowing me to be a part of this project.

And to everyone in the Healing GP group who shares their own stories and tips to keep us all inspired.

# NOTES

www.ingramcontent.com/pod-product-compliance
Lightning Source LLC
Chambersburg PA
CBHW050124280326
41933CB00010B/1232